THE LITTLE CANCER BOOK
FOR PATIENTS

WHAT YOU SHOULD KNOW

BRIAN PLANTS, MD

The Little Cancer Book for Patients
www.AskTheCancerDoc.com
© 2020 Brian Plants, MD

The *Ask the Cancer Doc* logo is a trademark of RadOncHelpline, LLC.

First Edition

PRINT ISBN: 978-1-7345412-0-5

Table of Contents

DISCLAIMER

- Dr. Plants does *not* provide medical services or practice medicine by answering questions.

- He is neither diagnosing any disease nor treating any disease or illness by providing educational services through this book or the *Ask the Cancer Doc* website.

- No specific or individual personal health information is collected or stored as a result of any online or telecommunication services.

- All services are for educational purposes only.

- Any medical decisions made by our customers as a result of the information in this book or medical outcomes relating to any interaction with this book or the *Ask the Cancer Doc* website are the sole responsibility of the customer.

- Dr. Plants and any other entity affiliated with the *Ask the Cancer Doc* website assumes no responsibility of any kind relating to information discussed, sent, received, or shared during any business transaction.

- We do *not* provide medical consultations or services and are not licensed to practice medicine in most states.

ACKNOWLEDGMENTS

To my Lord and Savior, Christ Jesus, from whom I draw each breath;

To my dad, Chester, for teaching me to properly apply "attitude" and "effort" and how to be a man;

To my mom, Sue, for always putting others before herself and showing me what love really means;

To my lovely wife, Betsy Plants, MD, my best friend, who was invaluable in the creation of this book (it would take another book to list all the ways);

To my two older children, Rachel and Jason, for applying just a small portion of their considerable skills to help with editing; my youngest son, Luke, for demonstrating what true faith and courage look like; and to all three for inspiring me to be a better man;

To my friend and coworker, Elise Stevens, FNP-BC, for her assistance with initial editing and for years of sharing her talents and love to those who are sick;

To J. A. Vargo, MD, one of the smartest, coolest, and all-around-nicest guys that I've ever met, for his knowledge and help editing some finer points of this book;

To all my coworkers for the years of support and help caring for many thousands of patients—you make a difference that truly matters.

To all those who suffer or have a loved one who suffers with the dreadful disease of cancer.

FOREWORD

The purpose of this booklet is to help patients and their families understand a cancer diagnosis and to briefly introduce some common cancer treatment options. It is not intended to be a medical text for physicians or other medical professionals, although they may also benefit from it. Patients face the daunting task of sorting through mountains of medical literature and clicking through an endless stream of websites to find accurate information about cancer. My goal is to share general principles and explanations with you which my patients have found helpful over the years. As an oncologist, writing sweeping generalizations on these complex topics in an easy-to-understand way is more challenging than you may assume; I can think of an exception to almost every sentence I have written, so it is important to speak to your doctor concerning the issues discussed herein as well. Nevertheless, this does not diminish the value of clearly stating some basic concepts that may help patients wade through the mire. Some of these principles were trained into me through 13 years of formal training post-high school, others were acquired by on-the-job-training, referred to as the "practice of medicine".

Many of the topics that we will discuss are very complex, so I have attempted to explain them in simple, comprehensible terms without overlooking the main issue of how it relates to cancer patients. A glossary is included at the end of this booklet to briefly explain some of the less common terms that are mentioned. I could not help myself from including some pearls of wisdom and encouragement for patients and families—pearls that have become ingrained in my explanation of these topics after nearly two decades of practicing radiation oncology. It is my intention that you may be helped in some way by these words. In the chapters that follow, I want to help you understand the big picture and what to expect. *Part I* of this book will explain *Cancer Basics*, while *Part II* addresses some of the particulars of the most common *Specific Types of Cancer*. I hope these pages will help you learn what cancer is, how it spreads, what tests you may need, and common ways to treat it. There are many more specifics regarding surgery, chemotherapy, immunotherapy, radiation therapy, research trials, and basic cancer statistics that can be uncovered online. If you are inclined to learn more, I *highly recommend* the websites of the **American Cancer Society** at http://www.cancer.org and the **National Cancer Institute (NCI)** at https://www.cancer.gov or you can contact me directly at http://www.AskTheCancerDoc.com.

PROLOGUE

TRAGEDY STRIKES US ALL

A loud crash shook the house, followed by deafening silence. My first thought was that one of my three kids had knocked the TV off the wall, and I yelled downstairs, "What was that?" An uneasy three-second-pause was followed by a feeling in my gut that propelled my feet towards the stairs. I passed my wife as we ran down the steps only to see my younger son, Luke, lying unconscious on the floor. He looked as if he was asleep, but there was blood on the beige carpet next to his head. I felt sick to my stomach. Having seen many trauma patients in my training, I was familiar with setting aside my feelings as I assessed the situation as quickly and accurately as possible—but this time, it was my son. I could feel my heart beating in my neck and it seemed as though I was in a dream. It was surreal—as if time had stopped. I tried to process what my eyes were seeing. As I entered the room, I saw my middle son, Jason, put down the weight that only moments before had pinned his younger brother to the floor. Somehow, he had managed to lift it off him. Their older sister, Rachel, was in shock, standing frozen and silent a couple of steps away.

Initially, I couldn't determine where the blood originated from—his body was lying on his right side and seemed intact. When I knelt beside him, I notice some blood pooled in his left ear and around the openings of his nose. He had a weak pulse, but he was not breathing, and I wasn't about to wait for an ambulance. I scooped him up as we all scrambled to the car. I handed him over to my wife, Betsy, in the backseat as I drove off our hill and across the bridge toward the hospital. Fortunately, we live near the best trauma center in our state and there was no traffic. My mind was racing with doubts about whether I was doing the right thing or if I should've called 9-1-1. Only later did my wife tell me that our baby had turned an ashen, blue-gray color and she had to give him mouth-to-mouth breathing. She still felt his pulse, but without help that wouldn't last for long. I pulled right up to the Emergency Department, took him into my arms, and raced inside. The hospital staff immediately went into action and had him intubated and ventilated within eight minutes from the time of the crash. It happened so fast that I didn't have time to be scared.

As I handed off my little boy to the professionals, I looked to my wife to see if she and the other kids were alright. We were pacing back and forth and that's when I really started to worry. The sick feeling in my gut intensified and my mind raced. Betsy had enough sense to call our family and a couple of close friends. I went to the CT and MRI scans with Luke and then to the ICU where he was on a ventilator for many days. A neurosurgeon, one of my colleagues, placed an intracranial pressure sensing device, called a "bolt", in his skull to measure the pressure of the brain. It took a few days for the swelling in his brain to reach a maximum and then slowly begin to decrease. For a while, surgery on the brain to relieve pressure was the main concern. When I finally arrived home from the hospital two days later, I realized how heavy the weight machine really was. It had stood about seven feet above the floor and weighed several hundred pounds. With my son's dried blood still on my T-shirt from the accident, I bent over to deadlift one end of the machine as Jason had done. I estimate that it was at least 200-250 pounds—quite a feat for a 10-year-old boy to accomplish even with the aid of adrenaline.

We all knew it was bad, but it wasn't until a few months later that my trauma surgeon friend told me *just how bad*. Luke had been diagnosed with Diffuse Axonal Injury (DAI), a form of traumatic brain injury that has a mortality rate of over 90% and those that survive usually have serious, life-long problems even after rehabilitation. To everyone's surprise, Luke went from not being able to feed himself to playing middle school soccer, basketball, and track. Despite a tremor that makes it difficult to write, his handwriting has greatly improved, and electronic tablets help him take notes and complete assignments. Thanks to his ever-amazing mom and many supportive teachers and friends, he did not even miss a grade of school. At church, some refer to my son as a "walking miracle"—I think he is too. There will always be ramifications from the accident, but watching him slowly recover, grow, and adapt to new challenges encourages my soul in a way that few things have in my life. Whether it be from excellent medical care or divine intervention, I believe God was watching over his recovery and the welfare of my family. As odd as it may be, I never experienced complete contentment until I sat in the ICU with my youngest son. The Bible speaks of a "peace that passes all understanding" and I can assure you that it is real. I hope that with whatever you may be going through, you too can experience this level of peace.

While I have not been diagnosed with cancer, my son's traumatic brain injury helped me relate to some of the fear, frustration, and suffering of my own cancer patients. Fear, primarily, of an unknown future. Frustration with a process that we cannot control. Suffering experienced by our bodies and felt in our souls. Whether it be from trauma or cancer, a bad diagnosis impacts us and everyone around us. It may never be welcomed, but it does help us to focus on what is really important. It forces us to reexamine our lives and relationships. Hopefully, it reminds us that each day brings opportunities to be kind and to share in meaningful moments with the ones we love.

PART ONE

CANCER BASICS

CHAPTER ONE

WHAT DID THE DOCTOR JUST SAY?

If you or a loved one has been diagnosed with cancer, you will have questions. What did the doctor just say? How did this happen? What do I do now? Where do I go for help? These are good questions. I hope to help you cut through the noise, dispel false information, and guide you through the diagnosis of cancer without being too technical or finding ourselves lost in the weeds.

So, what do you do when a doctor says you have cancer? First, you take a deep breath...and then another...and another... Give yourself a break. It is going to take a while to process what you've been told, what it means, and how it will affect you and your loved ones. The journey that has been thrust upon you may take many weeks, months, or even years to sort through. Allow yourself to experience this process. Fighting cancer is like being forced to ride an emotional roller coaster you never stood in line for. Overwhelmed by uncertainty and fear, it is not unusual to suffer from temporary bouts of denial, anger, depression, numbness, and panic. I've been told that one can be glad, mad, and sad all in the same day or even feel nothing at all.

The shock of a cancer diagnosis can cause some patients to experience decision-making paralysis. Find a trusted friend, family member, or confidant to help you process the things your doctor is going to tell you. While it is normal to have these feelings, at some point, you must move into problem-solving mode. You may not be offered much time to make medical decisions, usually just a few days, so don't be afraid to ask for help. The doctor that told you about the cancer will advise you on what to do next and probably make a referral to a cancer specialist. Some patients also find it valuable to assemble their own team of helpers; which may include family, friends, counselors, and spiritual support, in addition to their team of medical professionals. There are also support groups and online resources—but be careful. The internet is full of both good and bad information. You might consider asking your family doctor which cancer doctor (oncologist) he or she recommends for consultation regarding your type of cancer. When you go to a consultation with an oncologist, bring one or two family members or friends to listen, take notes, and ask questions. It is important, however, that whomever you bring can deal with difficult adult conversations. Although the vast amount of information online can be intimidating, it may also help to learn about possible treatment options from credible websites like those I cite in the Foreword.

CHAPTER TWO

WHO ARE ALL THESE DOCTORS?

Prior to a cancer diagnosis, when a patient first complains of symptoms, his or her family doctor usually asks questions, performs an exam, and may order some tests. If your family doctor suspects a cancer, he/she may refer you to a surgeon for a biopsy (i.e. surgery to sample a piece of tissue from the tumor). However, sometimes biopsies are performed by interventional radiologists (i.e. CT-guided biopsy), gastroenterologists (i.e. colonoscopy with biopsy for tumors of the gut), or other types of doctors. The tissue from the biopsy is reviewed under a microscope by a different type of doctor, called a pathologist. If cancer cells are seen under the microscope, then the pathologist confirms the diagnosis of cancer and reports this information back to the surgeon. It is the surgeon's duty to inform the patient whether they have cancer or not and, if appropriate, make a referral to an oncologist. At this point, the surgeon may order additional tests or medical scans to determine the size and location of the cancer or to look for other problem areas.

Following diagnosis, your surgeon may also refer you to an oncologist for additional evaluation. Oncologists are cancer doctors that specialize in treating different types of cancer and include medical oncologists and radiation oncologists. A medical oncologist prescribes treatments in the form of medicines, such as chemotherapy, hormonal therapy, immunotherapy, and/or biological therapy to treat cancers. A radiation oncologist is a different type of cancer specialist that uses radiation (X-ray) treatments to treat or kill cancers. Large cancer centers, like those affiliated with the National Comprehensive Cancer Network (NCCN), often recommend that cancer patients be evaluated by a multidisciplinary team (i.e. all three types of cancer doctors—surgeon, radiation oncologist, and medical oncologist) to discuss which tests and treatments are appropriate for your situation. Each physician contributes a slightly different perspective in the decision-making process, but treatment decisions should be based on accepted standards of care.

Each year, a wide range of cancer specialists review new therapies and the best cancer treatments that are currently available for each type of cancer and publish their recommendations in nationally recognized treatment guidelines, like those of the NCCN. Cancer treatment guidelines for oncologists are like cookbooks for a chef. There are many guidelines and other sources of information from research trials and medical literature that help cancer doctors to recommend the right treatment for you. It is important to remember that patients' cases are not always straightforward and there are often exceptions that make decisions more difficult. Sometimes, cancer cases are presented to a "tumor board", where a group of cancer specialists review a patient's medical records—including pathology slides, radiology images, and laboratory results to collaborate on the best plan of treatment. While national cancer treatment guidelines do give specific direction, they are not enough to cover every possible scenario that oncologists face. Flexibility and professional judgment are necessary to modify treatment recommendation for the specifics of each patient's case. Returning to the cooking analogy, a good oncologist is like a good chef that knows what ingredient to substitute in case the pantry is a bit bare or what temperature setting to place his particular oven because one of the heating elements isn't working properly and runs a bit cooler than most. It is with these complicated cases that a multidisciplinary team of doctors can really be helpful.

CHAPTER THREE

WHAT TESTS DO I NEED?

Your records are usually sent to the oncologist before your oncology appointment, but all patients are asked to fill out additional paperwork prior to the consultation. Despite seeming redundant, it is necessary to help ensure that no important information has been overlooked. Screening tests, like colonoscopies, mammograms, CT scans for heavy smokers, and PSA blood tests, are done to find cancers before patients have any clinical symptoms. Symptoms of cancer may include some of the following: unexplained weight loss, swollen "glands" (these are really lymph nodes), fever, sore throat, earache, headache, cough, pain, fatigue, and other general symptoms. When a patient presents with symptoms like those listed, the doctor usually performs a history and physical exam and may order some blood tests. One of the most common blood tests, a complete blood count (CBC) blood test is used to check the *oxygen-carrying* red blood cells, the *infection-fighting* white blood cells, and the *blood-clotting* platelets. If these tests are abnormal, other tests may be ordered. Blood tests to screen for some cancers may include PSA (prostate specific antigen for prostate cancer), CEA (carcinoembryonic antigen for colon cancer), CA-125 (cancer antigen 125 for ovarian cancer), or other tumor markers.

Unfortunately, most lab tests are nonspecific and are used by doctors as clues rather than giving a specific diagnosis. Some of these tumor markers can be used to monitor the effectiveness of treatment. Unfortunately, most cancer types don't have reliable tumor markers to measure.

After some initial tests identify an area of concern, the only way to confirm that a person has cancer is for a surgeon to sample, or biopsy, some of the suspicious tissue. Taking a piece of the tumor can be done with a needle, a core biopsy, or an open biopsy. Some biopsies are done with the aid of ultrasound or CT guidance to make sure the tumor is sampled properly. Even though it may be frustrating, it is not unusual for biopsies to be inadequate or inconclusive. Even if the tumor was properly sampled, tumors are often necrotic (rotten) in the middle and the tissue sampled may not be able to be identified.

As discussed above, the tissue from a biopsy is sent to a doctor that specializes in looking at cells and tissue under a microscope, called a pathologist. The pathologist uses stains and special dyes to determine the type of cancer and assigns it a grade. Tumor grade describes the cancer's level of aggressiveness and its likelihood of spread as low, medium, or high. The pathology results usually take about 2–7 days to obtain a final diagnosis. The pathologic review is critical and must be done properly because treatment recommendations will depend upon the results. The pathologist will inform the surgeon of the results, who, in turn, notifies the patient and usually makes a referral to an oncologist.

In addition to your initial medical tests, your oncologist is probably going to order even more tests before deciding on which treatment plan is best suited to your situation. To make the best decisions, oncologists need several important pieces of information—the patient's symptoms, biopsy results, medical imaging (scans), and clinical examination.

While some medical scans, like a CT (computed tomography, or CAT) scan, may have been done during the workup prior to your biopsy, more scans will likely be needed after your diagnosis to assess the current size and location of the tumor and whether it has spread to other parts of the body. Some common medical scans used today include CT scans, MRI (magnetic resonance imaging) scans, PET/CT (positron emission tomography/computed tomography) scans, and bone scans. CT scans use 3-dimensional X-rays, are found in most hospitals, show very good anatomical details of most organs and lymph nodes, and can be done quickly. MRI scans use magnetic waves to show exquisite detail of some soft tissues and neurologic tissue, like the brain; but MRIs are slow, noisy, and uncomfortable due to the small aperture (i.e. opening) that can cause claustrophobic symptoms in some patients. PET/CT and bone scans are both nuclear medicine tests that use a very low dose of radioactive liquid tracer injected into the blood so it can travel to various organs of the body. Bone scans are good at seeing if cancer has spread (or metastasized) to the bones, but PET/CT can do that and much more. Since cancer cells grow quickly, they typically consume large amounts of sugar (glucose) and a PET/CT is helpful because it shows where sugar (glucose) is being used in the body. PET/CTs are helpful in finding where tumors may have spread, however, they can also light up falsely from other causes, like infections (pneumonia), old traumas (fractures), inflammation, normal physiology, diabetes, etc. Your doctor can help explain what areas on a PET/CT are likely to be cancer or not. False-positive areas of enhancement may mislead oncologists resulting in an overestimation of tumor spread. Some tumors may also be overlooked because the brain, heart, kidneys, bladder, and other normal tissues enhance normally and may mask small underlying tumors. Several different tests are usually necessary during staging workups because each test has different strengths and weaknesses. Oncologists need multiple tests because one test cannot see everything.

A major challenge is that tumors can't even be detected until they are at least 1/4 inch or bigger. The lower limit of detection on even the best medical imaging scans is about 6-10 millimeters (mm). The frightening part comes when we realize that about a million cancer cells can fit on the tip of a ballpoint pen. By the time the doctor sees a spot on a scan, the tumor would have over 100 million cells or so. Regarding the timing of medical scans, it is also important to be aware of how the cancer's biology and growth are affected by cancer treatment. Rather than repeatedly ordering medical imaging during treatment, scans are usually done after several months or after completing certain phases of the treatment to determine whether the tumor has responded or not. The reason is that there is a lag time between cancer cell death and the time it takes for the cancer's dead carcass to shrink and scar over. An exception to this slow shrinkage is in very sensitive tumors, like small cell lung cancer, testicular seminoma or various lymphomas, that dissolve quickly. We will discuss cancer biology in the next chapter.

CHAPTER FOUR

WHAT DOES IT MEAN TO HAVE CANCER?

If you don't understand what it means to have cancer, you are not alone. Most people lack a basic understanding of what cancer is, how it starts, and where it spreads, let alone possess a working knowledge of what to do about it. The word "cancer" strikes fear into the heart, and many cannot even bring themselves to speak the word aloud. I've even heard healthcare workers refer to the disease by the euphemism "CA" because the word itself is terrifying. Nevertheless, I believe that learning about one's adversary helps to develop a strategy for success and overcomes fear.

Cancer is not just one disease. Cancer is complicated. It is a disease as individualized as each of us. There are hundreds of types of cancer, and each cancer is unique because each patient is unique. The type of cancer depends on where it started in the body or, more specifically, the type of cell from which it originated. For example, a prostate cancer begins with a normal prostate cell that malfunctions and begins to grow out of control. Breast cancer, lung cancer, and hundreds of other cancers generally start and spread in similar patterns. Despite the similarities of certain types of cancer, each is still one-of-a-kind. I have witnessed two different patients with the same cancer undergo the exact same treatment and have two totally different results. To understand why, we must look at how normal cells transform into cancer cells.

HOW DO DNA MUTATIONS CAUSE CANCER?

In the human body there are over 30 trillion cells. Each one is controlled by the cell's nucleus. The cell nucleus contains the genetic information, or blueprints of the cell, within the famous macromolecule—DNA. A basic principle of cell biology is that DNA is "transcribed" into RNA and then the RNA is "translated" into the proteins that do most of the work in cells. Cells make up tissues, tissues make up organs, and organs make up a human body. Cancer is a disease where the cells from one part of the body keep growing when they are not supposed to grow. The cancer cells multiply faster and more often than normal cells. Cell growth is ordinarily regulated by the DNA, but DNA can be damaged by mutations or copying errors as cells divide over time. A damaged DNA molecule causes a normal cell to become cancerous by turning off some of the checks and balances that prevent the cell from multiplying too often.

There are many different mutations that can damage DNA. Some mutations affect the cell's life expectancy, drastically lengthening it. Normal cells naturally die through a process of pre-programmed cell death, called apoptosis. This process is too complicated to fully explain here, but essentially, the DNA molecule is shortened a little bit each time normal cells divide. After a certain number of cell divisions, the DNA is depleted and too shortened to keep the cell alive any longer. However, if a cell can prevent the DNA ends from being shortened by a protein enzyme, called telomerase, the cell has a chance of becoming immortal, or growing indefinitely. Some mutations may also result in damage to part of the cell's defense mechanisms, like the proofreader genes that fix copying errors inside the cell's DNA, called tumor suppressor genes. These genes help regulate cell growth, while other mutations may cause an imbalance in proteins that cause cell migration and help cancer cells spread to other parts of the body. When a cancer spreads through the lymph nodes or blood, it is called a metastasis. These unwelcome changes are just a few of the many missteps that cells undergo to become a cancer cell. Other mutations allow cancer cells to recruit and grow new blood vessels to supply more nutrients and oxygen to nourish the tumor and allow for faster growth. Still other cancer mutations knock out parts of the immune system to prevent the body from finding and stopping the cancer. If this sounds like biological warfare, that's because this is exactly what it is, and your body has been winning your entire life. Sometimes though, the body needs a little help.

How Do I Develop Mutations and What Are My Risk Factors?

Despite what we know about risk factors for cancers, most of the time there doesn't seem to be a single obvious thing people do which causes cancer. Risk factors become apparent when analyzing thousands of patients, but when speaking to patients one at a time, I cannot usually discern an identifiable cause. Developing a cancer seems to have less to do with diet, exercise, and lifestyle than most people think. Although there is no doubt that smoking is an obvious lifestyle choice that affects a person's risk of developing a cancer, it is also true that most smokers don't get lung cancer.

Don't misunderstand—please don't smoke. Smoking greatly increases the risks of COPD, heart attacks, strokes, and other diseases. Smoking also decreases the cure rate of cancer treatments by increasing the risk of recurrence, reducing wound healing, and increasing the chance of side effects from treatment. Some other risk factors associated with normal cells mutating into cancer cells include chemical exposure, advanced age, weight gain, alcohol, and genetics. Nevertheless, most cancer mutations are random, and its cause does not come with an explanation. Cancer runs in some families, so there must be some genetic predisposition to developing cancer but, for now, most of these genetic risks are undetectable. Some rare mutations, like BRCA 1 & 2 gene mutations in breast cancer patients, have been discovered, but most of the genetic factors that contribute to developing a cancer have not yet been identified. I think most people assume that if they have a cancer then something went wrong—biologically maybe, but not necessarily in a practical sense. I view cancer as a part of life, whether we like to admit it or not. An unpleasant fact of life is that if we are breathing, we are at risk of developing various cancers. It is even possible for a person to have more than one type of cancer over their lifetime. I've treated many patients with a history of two different and unrelated cancers. It is not uncommon to be completely cured of one cancer and then develop an entirely different cancer years later. If a previously treated cancer re-grows, or newly growing tumors are discovered during the first 5-10 years after a cancer treatment, it is more likely to be a recurrence of the original cancer, but not always. Some "recurrences" may be totally different cancers, particularly if they appear more than 10-15 years after the original cancer. Treatment options for a new cancer are often very different than treatments for tumors that have been secretly hibernating and begin to regrow months or years later.

I recall taking care of a gentleman that developed four totally separate cancers over a 25-year period and beat them all. He survived cancers of the colon, larynx, and two different types of lung cancer. He was treated with a variety of combinations of surgery, chemotherapy, and radiation. It is probably safe to assume that he carried some unknown, genetic predisposition to developing cancer, but he also continued to smoke heavily for decades. Despite all this, he died of liver failure from a long history of alcohol abuse—not from cancer. He is proof that we should never underestimate a person's future because we often don't know how things might turn out. Nevertheless, oncologists attempt to group cancers into categories with similar characteristics so that we can recommend the most effective treatments.

The best way to classify cancers is to identify the type of cell from which they originated. Before birth, all cells of the body were developing from one of three types of cells—ectoderm, mesoderm, or endoderm. Tumors that originate from cells of the middle layer (called the mesoderm) are a rare type of cancer called a sarcoma; however, most tumors originate from cells that make up the skin (the ectoderm) or the lining of body organs (the endoderm). These cells can transform into cancers known as carcinomas. Carcinomas are classified into several different groups—the most common being adenocarcinomas and squamous cell carcinomas. According to the National Cancer Institute (NCI) definition, adenocarcinomas are "cancers that begin in glandular (secretory) cells. Glandular cells are found in tissue that lines certain internal organs and makes and releases substances in the body, such as mucus, digestive juices, or other fluids. Most cancers of the breast, pancreas, lung, prostate, and colon are adenocarcinomas." The NCI defines squamous cell carcinomas as cancers that "are found in the tissue that forms the surface of the skin, the lining of the hollow organs of the body, and the lining of the respiratory and digestive tracts. Most cancers of the anus, cervix, head and neck, and vagina are squamous cell carcinomas."[1] Some adenocarcinomas (like most breast and gastrointestinal cancers) usually require some type of surgery, but other adenocarcinomas (like prostate cancer) can often be cured with surgery or radiation therapy. Squamous cell carcinomas (like cancers of the larynx or anal canal) may be cured even without surgery using a combination of chemotherapy and radiation therapy as a part of an "organ-sparing" approach. Other parts of the body, like the brain or nervous system, have specialized cells that are prone to becoming other specific types of cancers.

How Can My Cancer Spread?

A tumor is an abnormal lump of cells that can be seen or palpated (felt with the fingers) anywhere in the body. A tumor may be benign or malignant. A benign tumor is unlikely to spread to other areas and is generally not likely to cause death. Benign tumors should not be routinely referred to as a cancer, although there are a few exceptions. Benign tumors may still require treatment because they can push against other tissues causing damage and physical symptoms as they grow. Examples of benign tumors include a list of unfamiliar names like acoustic schwannomas, gastrointestinal stromal tumors (GISTs), lipomas, meningiomas, papillomas, pituitary adenomas, and other even more rare growths. A malignant tumor, called a cancer, is a group of cells from any organ of the body that can also grow into a lump of tissue, but can spread in three different ways. Cancer cells may spread directly to local tissues, regionally to nearby lymph nodes, and/or distantly to other organs that are far away in the body.

Are There Really Three Types of Spread?

Regardless of the type of cancer or where it started, cancer starts out as a single, microscopic cell that may grow and spread to other parts of the body in three different ways. The *first type of spread* is called **direct invasion**. This type of tumor growth pushes directly into nearby tissues and, depending on what organs are nearby, may cause pain, bleeding, fracture of bones, permanent nerve damage, neurological problems, or other symptoms. The *second type of spread* is called a **regional metastasis**. Regional spread is when tumor cells migrate to the surrounding area via the local lymphatic system to nearby lymph nodes. The lymphatic system is a network of low-pressure vessels, like small veins, that connect lymph nodes and help the body defend against infections. Tumor cells can invade the lymph vessels and use them as a pathway to travel in a relatively orderly fashion from one lymph node to the next. Some reports have shown that certain cancers may "skip" a lymph node in 15-25% of patients[1,2]. The *third type of spread* is called **distant metastasis**, or **hematologic spread**, and occurs when tumor cells travel through the bloodstream. After cancer cells invade the blood, they travel through arteries and veins and can spread long distances to anywhere in the body. Once they've spread, these metastatic cells can begin to infiltrate the tissues in these new areas and attract new blood vessel growth to help them grow and spread further. Where a cancer spreads depends on the type of cancer, the percentage of blood flow to that area, and other factors. Distant metastasis most commonly involves the lung, liver, bone, and brain because these organs receive a majority of the body's blood flow. It may surprise you to know that cancer cells can spread while causing few, if any, symptoms. Others may experience vague symptoms that are hard to pinpoint or difficult to explain, such as general malaise, fatigue, bloating, weight loss, fevers, and more.

CHAPTER FIVE

WHAT ARE MY CHANCES OF BEING CURED?

The chance of being cured of cancer is linked to the stage of the cancer. A cancer's "stage" tells a cancer doctor where the tumor started, how big it is, how many different spots are involved, and what the chances of cure might be. To determine whether a cancer was found early or in an advanced stage, oncologists use the TNM staging system to describe how far along a cancer has spread. This classification system makes sense when you understand the three ways of spread described in the previous chapter. To determine the overall stage, we must explain what each letter of TNM means. The "T" stands for the primary "Tumor" (where it started) and describes the size of the initial tumor and how much it has directly invaded into nearby tissue (T1-small, T2-bigger, T3-bigger still, T4-biggest). The "N" stands for "Nodes", or regional lymph nodes (N0-no spread to regional lymph nodes, N1-a few lymph nodes involved, N2-3-many lymph nodes involved). The "M" stands for distant "Metastasis" (M0-no distant metastasis, M1- distant metastasis). The TNM stages are complicated, but when taken together allow a cancer to be assigned an overall stage grouping signified by the Roman numerals (I, II, III, or IV). There are many exceptions, but, Stage I and II tumors are small and localized, Stage III tumors have spread to the regional lymph nodes, and Stage IV tumors have usually spread to distant parts of the body through the bloodstream.

To dive a little deeper into cancer staging, it is necessary to realize that there are two types of staging— *clinical* and *pathologic*, depending on whether a "staging surgery" was used to obtain pathologic information. While a biopsy of some form is almost always required to diagnose cancer, a staging surgery often includes an attempt to completely remove the tumor and a surgical lymph node evaluation. For example, breast cancer may be diagnosed via a small core needle biopsy, but to determine the tumor's size and extent of spread requires a larger surgery, like a lumpectomy or mastectomy and some form of lymph node dissection. If you can't or don't have surgery to stage your cancer, you will be *clinically* staged to assign a *clinical* TNM stage and a *clinical* stage group using only physical exam and medical imaging scans. If you have surgery to stage your cancer, you will be *pathologically* staged and given a *pathologic* TNM stage and *pathologic* stage group. Since some tumors are too small to be seen on medical scans but may be seen under the microscopic exam following a staging surgery, the *pathologic staging* is more accurate. The downside of *pathologic staging* is that a staging surgery is more extensive than a biopsy and more invasive than a simple medical scan and some patients are unwilling or unable to undergo a full surgical evaluation.

CAN CANCER REALLY BE CURED?

Overall, more than half of my patients have been/are considered curable or cured. The word "cure" means that the cancer never comes back. Notice that I did not use the word "remission", which means that the cancer is not seen on a scan but may still be hiding and ready to return in the future. Cure rates are generally better with smaller tumors and tumors that have not spread, but there are exceptions. The staging system is important in estimating both the cure rate and life expectancy. Stage I cancers are cured most often, followed by Stage II, and then Stage III cancers. The actual cure rates vary dramatically based on the specific type of tumor and many other factors yet staging gives us a "ballpark" cure rate and helps to inform us as to which treatments are best. Unfortunately, tumors that have spread through the blood (M1) are considered stage IV and are often not curable; however, there are a few exceptions. For example, some Stage IV cancers—like lymphomas, testicular seminomas, and some other "sensitive" cancers, may be cured with chemotherapy and systemic treatments (even if they've spread throughout the body). There are other well-documented exceptions, such as in colon cancer patients with only a single distant metastasis to the liver. If surgically removed and chemotherapy is given, the long-term cure rate is around 25% (25 out of 100) when it should theoretically be zero[1]. More recent data using focal, high-dose radiation therapy for patients with spread through the blood (M1—Stage IV), but only a few distant metastasis (called oligo-metastasis) have also shown dramatic improvements in survival and tumor control, particularly when used in combination with new regimens of immunotherapy[2]. Unfortunately, these encouraging results are not the case for most Stage IV cancers.

To understand the relationship between cure rate and stage, it is important to recognize that despite all the recent advances in medical imaging, a medical scan cannot "see" or detect cancer cells until they are at least several millimeters in size (minimum 6-10 millimeters or a 1/4 inch even with the best tests). While that may sound small to some, we must realize that one millimeter of tumor consists of about one million cancer cells. Therefore, a 6-7-millimeter "spot" on a scan *may* be 6-7 million cancer cells. The problem is that there are many *normal* "spots" that appear on medical scans, such as cysts, scars, infections, or other benign "lesions" that mimic but are NOT cancer. (Again, benign "lesions" don't grow and spread, they usually just sit there and do nothing.)

Furthermore, if a group of tumor cells is smaller than 6-10-millimeters, it often won't even show up on medical scans. So, it is not uncommon for a patient to be diagnosed with a Stage I, II, or III cancer (i.e. no appearance of distant metastasis) only to find out months or years later that there were cancer cells (maybe even thousands of them) hiding elsewhere in the body all along that didn't show up on medical scans. In other words, the patient would have been staged with an M1 (Stage IV) cancer, but the cancer cells were too small to be seen on the medical scans. To be blunt, these "curable" patients had cancer cells that had already spread throughout the body [i.e. distant metastasis—M1 (Stage IV)] and were actually not likely to be curable even at the time of diagnosis, but neither the patient nor the doctor had any way of knowing. The cancer cells that had already spread were simply too small to detect. Had the metastasis been large enough to be seen on imaging tests, the patient would've been labeled Stage IV and likely told that cure was not likely possible.

So, how does an oncologist know that their patient doesn't *really* have an undetectable Stage IV cancer? How does a Stage I, II, or III patient *really* know if they "caught" the cancer before it spread through the blood? They can't—at least not immediately or in the short term. There is currently no way for modern medical scans to detect the spread of individual cancer cells. There are, however, new blood tests that are attempting to isolate individual cancer cells circulating in the bloodstream, but these tests are currently being studied and a topic of current research trials. Whether we like it or not, we must come to grips with the fact that cancer is sneaky, and our tests are far from perfect. At this time, we must continue to make treatment decisions based on the scans and medical information that we currently have available. The inability to see individual cancer cells or detect early spread is why oncologists must rely on staging guidelines and cancer statistics. We must lean on the lessons learned from the thousands of patients that have come before. It is important to understand that just because a person may be diagnosed with a cancer that is not likely to be curable, does not mean that he or she shouldn't be treated. Cancer treatments often extend the length and quality of life even if cure is not achievable. Ultimately, only time will differentiate the patients that were not curable from those that *really* have been cured.

Before we leave this chapter dealing with cure rates, please allow me to share some advances in cancer treatment that give us encouragement for the future. A reason to hope is modeled by our fight against Hodgkin's Disease, a type of lymphoma. Hodgkin's lymphoma had a cure rate of zero in the 1950's—it was universally fatal. With the advent of near total-body radiation therapy and early mustard-based chemotherapy in the 1960's, about 50% of patients survived, albeit with serious side effects. Advances in chemotherapy in the 1970's improved cure rates to the 70% range. With the combination of modern chemotherapy, small-field (focal) radiation, PET-CT imaging, and other advances, the cure rate of Hodgkin's Disease is around 85-90% today with much less long-term toxicity and fewer side effects[2]. Those are impressive results in half a century. Unfortunately, tumors like glioblastoma of the brain, adenocarcinoma of the pancreas, and others are more difficult to cure. Progress is slow, but recent advances in genetics and targeted biologic therapy are very promising. Fortunately, current statistics indicate that, overall, well over half to two-thirds of cancer patients did "catch" their cancer before it spread and ***are curable.***

CHAPTER SIX

SO, HOW DO WE TREAT IT?

After helping thousands of patients journey from cancer diagnosis to treatment and recovery, I am still amazed at the prevalence of misinformation about cancer. Surprising to many patients, most healthcare professionals are not trained to know much about cancer diagnosis or treatment. Cancer decision-making can be very complicated—sometimes even for experts. In today's era of information overload, it requires considerable knowledge, experience, and skill to sort through vast amounts of information to make accurate and informed decisions. Nationally recognized treatment guidelines, results of cancer research, and collaboration with other physicians form the basis of how oncologists make treatment recommendations. In this chapter, we will discuss the main pillars of modern cancer treatments, namely—surgery, chemotherapy, biological therapy, and radiation therapy.

TELL ME ABOUT SURGERY

Surgery is an invasive procedure that physicians perform using instruments to investigate or treat a disease or injury. Most cancer patients undergo some type of surgery for diagnosis, treatment, or both. Surgery may be only a small biopsy used for diagnosis or a large cancer surgery to remove the tumor and nearby lymph nodes for definitive treatment. Contrary to some patient's first instincts, more surgery is not always better. Today, less drastic surgery and organ-sparing techniques allow for better cures with fewer side effects. The edges of the surgical specimen, called the surgical margins, are evaluated under the microscope by the pathologist to determine if any tumor cells remain after surgery. As previously described, cancer cells are too small to be seen with the naked eye and even with a microscope can be difficult to see. When cutting out a tumor, it is important to know that tumor cells grow outward with finger-like projections away from the mass. These "fingers" or "roots" can be like weeds. All the tumor's roots must be removed, or the cancer will simply regrow. It is important to cut out or kill any microscopic tumor cells to have the best chance at a cure. In early stage cancers, surgery may be all that is needed but there are many factors to consider. Depending on the diagnosis and stage of the cancer, chemotherapy and/or radiation therapy may also be given before or after surgery.

There are several types of surgeons depending on where the tumor is in the body. Tumors of the brain call for a neurosurgeon; head & neck, an ENT; chest, a cardiothoracic surgeon; belly, a general surgeon; urinary tract, a urologist; and female organs, a gynecologic oncologist (GYN Onc). Interestingly, a GYN Onc is the only surgeon that is dually trained to both perform surgery and deliver chemotherapy for cancers. Regardless of the type of surgeon, I recommend that you find a doctor with considerable experience and training in the type of surgery that you need and don't be afraid to ask questions. In general, surgeries may be open, laparoscopic, or robotic. Open surgeries have larger incisions and allow for more extensive surgery, such as extensive lymph node dissections. Laparoscopic or robotic surgeries have smaller incisions (<1 inch), use a camera, and report less blood loss and pain, thus allowing quicker recoveries. A modern trend in surgery is to remove less tissue with the goal of fewer side effects, such as lymphedema (swelling of the extremity). A good example of less surgery being preferred over larger surgeries is the use of the sentinel lymph node dissection in breast cancer patients. Traditionally, breast surgeons were trained for decades to remove 10-20 lymph nodes from the axilla (armpit area), called a complete axillary dissection, but recent research has proven equal or better results with the sentinel lymph dissection, whereby only 1–2 lymph nodes are removed from the axilla.

Prior to any major surgery, you can expect to undergo preoperative examinations, called preadmission testing, to make sure that you are fit enough for the procedure. Some common tests include a stress test to check your heart, pulmonary function tests (PFTs) to test your lungs, and blood work to test your kidneys. Surgery will require the use of intravenous lines (IVs) and some form of anesthesia. Afterward, you may need temporary plastic drains, dressings, and physical therapy before you can be discharged from the hospital. Remember to ask your surgeon how long your hospital stay should last as well as any other questions about these issues before surgery. A week or two after surgery, the pathologist will report the final results of the microscopic analysis of the tumor and lymph nodes. Specifically, the pathology report should spell out what kind of cancer was removed, its size, grade of aggressiveness, and whether the surgical margins were positive or negative. Contrary to how it sounds, a negative margin is a good thing. A negative (or clear) margin means that (according to the pathologist) all the tiny, microscopic roots of the tumor were completely removed during surgery. A positive margin means that some tumor remains inside the patient because at least one root of tumor is seen to extend all the way to the edge of where the surgeon cut the specimen. A close margin usually means that the roots of the tumor were removed with only one to two millimeters to spare, but it is still debatable in certain types of cancer as to whether this has a different outcome than a negative margin; in other words, how negative does negative need to be? This information from surgery is critical in assigning a final *"pathologic stage"* to the patient's tumor. As we previously mentioned, the pathologic stage is more accurate than the clinical stage that is only based on preoperative scans which estimate the size and extent of the tumor. Further treatment recommendations will be based on the pathologic stage. Make sure you ask for a copy of the pathology report to look for negative margins and whether tumor involved lymph nodes. Note: It is a good idea to keep copies of all your medical records and be able to let subsequent physicians know the results of your tests.

A major surgery may be avoided in some cancers, such as leukemias, lymphomas, and small cell lung cancers, that only require a biopsy because these are so sensitive to chemotherapy that extensive surgery does more harm than good. Other tumors, like squamous cell carcinomas of the larynx or anal canal, are so sensitive to a combination of chemotherapy and radiation that organ-sparing (i.e. leaving your organs intact in your body) is achievable without the need for surgery and the cure rates are just as good. Sometimes, large cancer surgeries may also be avoided in palliative situations where the goal is to maximize quality of life or make people comfortable. Surgeries with close or positive margins have higher rates of local recurrence and may benefit from further surgery or postoperative radiation therapy to kill any residual cancer cells that may be left inside the patient. Nevertheless, it is critical to understand that even under a microscope tumor spread can be easily missed. As I stated before, even with today's best medical imaging scans, we cannot see individual tumor cells—

that requires a microscope. After treatment, follow-up scans may be normal (some synonyms for normal are "clean", "clear", "negative", "in remission", and "stable") but neither you nor your doctor should be overly confident in these early scans. Some doctors use the word remission to let the patient know that their tumor has responded well to treatment, but remission does not mean the same as cure. Remission means that a tumor was treated, usually with chemotherapy, and is no longer seen on an imaging scan. Cure means that the cancer was completely killed and never comes back. Many patients in remission are not cured because microscopic "seeds" of tumor usually take months or years to grow large enough to be seen on medical scans. Only until a patient has been around for a few years with many normal scans do I even begin to consider using the word "cure". During the first few years, I interpret normal scans to my cancer patients as "cautiously optimistic". Unfortunately, many patients put too much trust in the imaging scans and may think they are cured only to be profoundly disappointed if a new spot of cancer appears on a scan two to three years down the road. It is good to rejoice over a good report, but be aware that individual tumor cells are too small to be seen and expectations should be tempered for the first few years after cancer treatments. Overall, techniques with surgery, pathology, and adjuvant treatments that may come after surgery, such as chemotherapy and radiation therapy, have dramatically improved in recent years and more people are cured and survive longer than ever before.

CHEMOTHERAPY: POISON OR MEDICINE?

Chemotherapy doctors, called medical oncologists, use drugs to treat cancer. In a way, chemotherapy is both a medicine and a poison. The goal is to heal the patient by poisoning the cancer. Chemotherapy attacks actively growing cells by damaging the cell's DNA and preventing it from dividing properly. Chemotherapy drugs also block specific proteins that cancer cells use to signal abnormal growth. They are taken up by both good and bad cells that are actively growing, and they cause a disruption in the cell cycle that results in cell death. Tumor cells are more affected by chemotherapy than normal cells because they are growing more quickly (tumors have an accelerated growth rate) and take up more of the drug as raw material needed for cell growth. I call this phenomenon the "hungry mouse" model. For example, when a pesky mouse is lurking around your house, one way to kill it is with a mouse poison called De-con. If the mouse is hungry, it will eat lots of poison and die; however, if the mouse just ate a big chunk of cheese then it may not want to eat your poisonous trap and will go on to live another day. Just like the hungry mouse, chemotherapy works better in fast growing tumors. The same principle is generally true for radiation therapy. Despite the obvious downside of fast-growing tumors spreading faster, one silver lining about fast growing tumors is that they often shrink faster; think hungry mouse—it dies quickly from eating the poison.

While chemotherapy has different side effects depending upon the drug, it is generally true that faster growing cells are more affected than less active cells. Unfortunately, rapidly growing normal cells, like the stomach lining, hair, fingernails, and bone marrow cells, are also affected by chemotherapy resulting in side effects like nausea, hair and nail loss, and a decrease in blood counts. It is very challenging to design a drug that targets just the bad cells. Targeted drug therapy is the holy grail in oncology, but cancer cells are good at hiding among normal cells. Think about trying to kill the weeds in your yard. If you spray weed-killer on your grass to kill a few pesky weeds, you end up with a brown spot of dirt because you killed all the grass too. Certain weed-killers specifically target the weeds but don't kill your grass. New biologic agents and immunotherapies use specific proteins, called antibodies, on the outside of cancer cells to specifically target and either directly kill the tumor or flag it for the body's immune system to devour. The trick is finding the right drug that matches a specific patient's cancer. There is tremendous potential for targeted systemic therapies, but medical research is just at the tip of the iceberg. Until more drugs are developed and more data is accumulated to guide us on when, where, and how, we must rely heavily on broad-coverage chemotherapies like capecitabine, carboplatin, cisplatin, docetaxel, doxorubicin, 5-fluorouracil (5FU), gemcitabine, paclitaxel, temozolomide, vincristine, etc.

Most chemotherapy treatments are given on an outpatient basis (in the doctor's office or hospital outpatient department), but some might require a hospital stay. Chemotherapy is usually given in multiple, small doses over several months rather than in one big dose. Multiple rounds of chemotherapy, called *cycles*, make up a *course* of chemotherapy. Doctors give chemotherapy in cycles, in which a period of treatment is followed by a period of rest to allow the body time to recover. Each cycle generally lasts for several weeks, but the amount of time between cycles and the number of cycles in each course depends on the type of chemotherapy. Most regimens are given about 3 weeks apart and last 3-4 months, but this can vary widely. Sometimes a patient may get one chemotherapy combination for several cycles and later switch to a different one if the first combination doesn't seem to be working. Most chemotherapy is a liquid that is given in intravenous (IV) form, but a few come in a pill form. For IV chemotherapy, a small round device, called a port, is surgically placed under the skin of the upper chest by a general surgeon to allow chemotherapy to be directly injected into the bloodstream. A port allows larger volumes of medicine to be delivered and provides IV (intravenous) access to prevent unnecessary needle sticks in the patient's arm every week. Traditionally, chemotherapy was given after surgery (adjuvant chemotherapy), but today many situations call for chemotherapy before surgery (neoadjuvant chemotherapy). Neoadjuvant chemotherapy often shrinks the tumor and allows doctors to see if the tumor responds to a chemotherapy. Smaller tumors are easier to surgically remove and may allow the surgeon to spare more normal tissue. Chemotherapy often increases the chances that the surgical margins will be negative, which leads to a higher chance of cure. Furthermore, giving chemotherapy before surgery allows medicine to get a head start on killing small tumor cells that may have spread to other parts of the body.

When undergoing chemotherapy, make sure to keep an updated list of all medications, vitamins, and supplements that you are taking. Remember to tell your doctor of any allergies or side effects from any previous medicines or chemicals that you've been exposed to in your lifetime. It is important to realize that vitamins and supplements are not regulated by the Food and Drug Administration (FDA) and the ingredients listed on the bottle are not necessarily the same chemicals or dosages of what is inside the bottle. Furthermore, even some natural substances may interfere with chemotherapy treatments so be sure to inform your medical oncologist of any medicine, supplement, or chemical that you are putting in your body.

Cancers and cancer treatments can cause side effects. Side effects are problems that occur when treatment affects healthy tissues or organs. Side effects from chemotherapy may be acute (i.e. mostly during or shortly after treatment) or late (i.e. months to years later). Acute side effects are typically temporary and may include fatigue, nausea, vomiting, diarrhea, hair loss, increased risk of bleeding or infection due to a decrease in blood counts, etc. (see Table 1). Keep in mind that side effects vary from person to person, even among those receiving the same treatment. Speak up about any side effects that you have, or changes you notice, so your health care team can treat or help you reduce these side effects.

Table 1. Chemotherapy Side Effects

- Anemia
- Appetite Loss
- Bleeding and Bruising (Thrombocytopenia)
- Cardiac Issues (Heart damage)
- Constipation
- Delirium
- Diarrhea
- Swelling (Edema)
- Fatigue
- Fertility Issues in Boys and Men
- Fertility Issues in Girls and Women
- Flu-Like Symptoms
- Hair Loss (Alopecia)
- Infection and Neutropenia
- Lymphedema
- Memory or Concentration Problems
- Mouth and Throat Problems
- Nausea and Vomiting
- Nerve Problems (Peripheral Neuropathy)
- Organ-Related Inflammation
- Pain
- Sexual Health Issues in Men
- Sexual Health Issues in Women
- Skin and Nail Changes
- Sleep Problems
- Urinary and Bladder Problems

To learn more about side effects or steps you can take to prevent or manage side effects see the National Cancer Institute (NCI) website at https://www.cancer.gov/about-cancer/treatment/side-effects.

Late side effects may occur after treatment and have a higher chance of being permanent and sometimes include infertility, damage to heart, lung, nerves or other organs, and even a small risk of a secondary cancer from the treatment. Ask your doctor or nurse which late side effects to watch for. See the section on Late Effects at https://www.cancer.gov/about-cancer/coping/survivorship/late-effects) to learn more. The benefits of chemotherapy must outweigh the risks for it to be part of the treatment plan. A final thought on chemotherapy: You can always quit if you don't like it, so if there is a good chance of a benefit, why not give it a try?

WHAT IS BIOLOGICAL THERAPY?

Medical oncologists are also experts in a newer class of drugs known as biological therapy. Biological therapy is a form of treatment that uses portions of the body's natural immune system to treat a disease. Some target specific molecules on cancer cells to destroy the cells, or it may target proteins that facilitate the growth of cancer cells. Others include a class of medicine, called immunotherapy, that enhance the body's immune system to fight cancers. Examples include medicines that are unfamiliar to most patients, such as laboratory-designed monoclonal antibodies (such as bevacizumab, cetuximab, trastuzumab, pertuzumab, and many others), interferon, interleukins, and colony-stimulating factors.

This new weapon against cancer enhances the body's ability to recognize cancers as an enemy by turning off parts of the body's normal system of checks and balances. Autoimmune diseases, like rheumatoid arthritis or lupus, occur when the body's immune system works in overdrive and attacks the normal tissues of the body. Immunotherapy works similarly to enhance the immune system to attack cancer cells, but an unwanted side effect may be that it also increases the chance of attacking some good tissues. While immunotherapy is more targeted than traditional chemotherapy, it is still nonspecific enough to affect many tissues in the body. Like chemotherapy, immunotherapy is a systemic treatment that may still cause side effects like skin redness, nausea, vomiting, diarrhea, cough, liver damage, abnormal hormone levels or more. Much more work needs to be done to figure out how and when to best use this new class of drugs.

Depending on the agent, biological therapies can be given by mouth, intravenously, or as an injection. Biological therapy is a very active and exciting area of cancer research. Interestingly, some recent data indicate that high-dose radiation therapy, like stereotactic body radiation therapy (SBRT), may further stimulate the immune system and enhance the cancer killing ability of some forms of immunotherapy.

HOW IS RADIATION THERAPY DIFFERENT?

More than half of all cancer patients receive radiation therapy at some point in their care. Radiation therapy is a cancer treatment that uses high-energy X-rays to kill cancer cells. Radiation therapy works by creating free radicals in the nucleus of cells that damage the cell's DNA. A normal cell's natural repair mechanisms fix almost all the damaged DNA in about 6 hours, but if the radiation damage builds up too fast (i.e. high doses per treatment) or if the cell tries to multiply through cell division (i.e. mitosis) too quickly, the cell may die before the damage can be repaired. Like chemotherapy, radiation works better on fast growing cells like cancer cells. Unlike chemotherapy that affects the entire body, radiation only affects the tissues within the radiation treatment field (i.e. the specific area where the radiation is being delivered). Radiation side effects are dependent on the amount of radiation given and the part of the body that is treated. When a person lies on the treatment table to receive external beam radiation, it does not get in the bloodstream nor does it make a person radioactive. After walking out of the treatment room, a patient may freely be near babies, children, and those that are pregnant without fear of harming others.

Radiation therapy can either be delivered externally (from a large machine) or internally (when a doctor places a small amount of radiation inside the body). Internal radiation (called brachytherapy) is less common and is typically used for some gynecologic or prostate cancers. Most radiation therapy patients receive high-energy X-rays via external radiation from a large machine called a linear accelerator that plugs into an electrical outlet. Radiation therapy is used to cure some patients and to relieve symptoms in others. If possible, the three goals of any cancer treatment are to cure, extend life, and/or improve quality of life. If attempting cure, we push patients through short-term discomfort to achieve a permanent cure. In patients that are not curable, our goal is to help the patient live longer and have a better quality of life. If we trade one day of misery during treatment for one good day after treatment is over—I wouldn't think that was a good trade. Everyone has a different way to view success, but if I could trade a month of temporary fatigue and sunburn for an extra 6-12 months of life—that makes more sense to me. Nevertheless, I can't promise all patients a longer life, but I may prevent pain, bleeding, a fracture, or some other serious tumor complication. At the end of the day, quality of life is most important and only the patient can decide what that really means.

Depending on the type of cancer, the size, and the location, radiation may best be given before (neoadjuvant), after (adjuvant), or in place of surgery. If given together (concurrently), the chemotherapy not only kills cancer cells on its own, but it also acts as a radiosensitizer, which means that it makes the radiation more effective. Unfortunately, concurrent chemo-radiation also increases the side effects on nearby normal tissues. Radiation given before surgery helps shrink tumors and achieve negative surgical margins. Radiation after surgery is used to kill any microscopic tumor cells that were missed and might be hiding around the operative bed or nearby lymph nodes. As stated earlier, it is important to realize that just because the surgical margins are negative does NOT mean that some tiny tumor cells weren't missed under the pathologist's microscope. It just means that the surgeon appeared to remove all the tumor cells. In smaller surgeries, like lumpectomy for breast cancer, most patients have up to a 30% chance of undetected tumor cells remaining just around the operative bed, even if margins were completely negative. It only takes one surviving cancer cell to regrow and repopulate the tumor. Radiation therapy is often used to kill any "roots" of tumor cells left behind and prevent tumor recurrence while also sparing the patient from the unnecessary side effects of larger surgeries. Another common purpose of radiation treatment is to relieve pain and suffering, called palliative radiation. Radiation therapy is particularly effective for bone metastasis and may diminish or eliminate pain from these areas of tumor spread.

Radiation treatments may be given by either photons, electrons, or protons. Most radiation centers use traditional X-rays, or photons, but some centers use proton therapy to minimize the low dose of radiation to surrounding tissues. Currently, there are no published results to show a benefit of proton therapy over modern treatments with X-rays (photons), but this is an active area of research. All radiation centers operate with the goal of delivering the correct dose of radiation to the cancer but keep the dose of radiation to the remainder of the body "As Low As Reasonably Achievable"—the ALARA principle. Don't let all the brand names of radiation equipment cause unnecessary confusion. There are many types of radiation machines available today and they are all amazingly accurate and reliable. Within the world of X-ray machines, linear accelerator brands include Varian's TrueBeam, Elekta's Synergy & Gamma Knife, Accuray's Tomotherapy & Cyberknife, and others. All modern radiation machines can deliver advanced forms of radiation like IMRT (Intensity-Modulated Radiation Therapy), VMAT (Volumetric-Modulated Radiation Therapy), IGRT (Image-Guided Radiation Therapy), and SBRT (Stereotactic Body Radiation Therapy).

Radiation is usually given over many treatments, or fractions, to allow the body to heal each day. Think of the tumor as an onion. If you've ever peeled an onion, you know that it has many layers. Each radiation treatment kills some cancer cells, like peeling a layer of the onion. Each treatment "peels" the tumor (onion) by another layer until finally killing the core of the tumor. If the cancer cells are killed before spreading elsewhere, then the patient may be cured—although you won't really know or confirm this until years later. Typically, radiation treatments last about 15 minutes per day and are delivered Monday through Friday, five days per week. The number of treatments can be as few as one treatment or as many as 35 treatments depending on the situation. Today, technology allows radiation to be delivered with fewer, more precise treatments. For small tumors, some patients may opt to receive one high-dose treatment known as *stereotactic radiosurgery (SRS)* or two to five high-dose treatments, called *Stereotactic Body Radiation Therapy (SBRT)*. These specialized treatments require advanced equipment using *Image-Guidance Radiation Therapy (IGRT)* to make sure that treatments are very precise (within one to two millimeters accuracy). These stereotactic treatments deliver doses of radiation so high that it is considered ablative, meaning that most cells in the high-dose area are killed (both tumor and normal cells). Therefore, stereotactic treatments must be limited to relatively small tumors (usually less than five centimeters). Most other types of radiation treatments are based on longstanding principles of radiation therapy that have been developed over the last 50-60 years. In traditional radiation therapy, treatments are given five days per week and typically last anywhere between two to seven weeks total. The amount of radiation dose is measured in a unit of dose called Gray (Gy) and can be given at rates of 1.8-2.0 Gy per day for traditional treatments all the way up to 24 Gy in a single *SRS* treatment. There are "in-between" regimens, referred to as *moderate hypofractionation*, that is a middle ground commonly used today in some cancers to give 3-4 Gy per day over 2–5 weeks.

A radiation oncologist uses data from your CT scan to create a 3-dimensional computer model of your body that is used to develop a specific radiation treatment plan for you. During the past twenty years, monumental advances in computer technology and software have allowed radiation to be delivered in ways that were previously not possible. For example, *Intensity-Modulated Radiation Therapy (IMRT)* uses complicated computer algorithms that optimize the best radiation plan from thousands of possible treatment options. In a practical sense, IMRT allows the radiation to "curve" around normal tissues and "paint" the dose on the tumor. The radiation beam doesn't really curve, the computer just allows us to "outflank" the tumor and break each radiation field into hundreds of "little fields", or beamlets, to deliver radiation from many different directions. A more recent advance, *Volumetric-Modulated Arc Therapy (VMAT)* delivers many little beamlets while the head of the linear accelerator is moving in 360-degree arcs around the patient. There are advantages and disadvantages to each technique, but VMAT can often deliver an elegant plan in just a couple of minutes each day. Today, almost all large cancer centers have modern radiation equipment capable of these radiation techniques.

The radiation process begins with a consultation with a radiation oncologist, a physician trained to design radiation treatments and to direct a team of healthcare professionals that deliver X-rays to treat cancers. The physician meets with the patient to decide which treatment is best and then designs a radiation plan to specifically fit each patient. Because each patient's anatomy is unique, a special CT scan is performed to map out the patient's anatomy while lying in the treatment position. This planning CT scan, called a simulation, is performed by certified Radiation Therapy Technologists (RTTs), referred to as radiation therapists. The CT simulation may last 20-30 minutes and usually involves the creation of some immobilization devices like a vacuum mold (think customized bean bag made from plastic or foam) or a plastic facemask for cancers of the head or neck. These immobilization devices help the patient comfortably lie still so the radiation will go to just the right spot every day. During this simulation procedure, lasers are used to help place marks on the skin with either an ink pen or a couple dots of permanent tattoo ink to allow a reproducible setup. This entire visit typically requires less than an hour and the data is sent to a special computer for treatment planning.

Simple plans can sometimes be done within a few days, but typical treatment plans usually require about 5-10 days to complete and check for quality assurance prior to starting treatment. During this time, the physician "draws" the tumor and other areas of concern on the images. Then radiation specialists, called medical dosimetrists, use computer software to create possible treatment plans using various beam angles and radiation modifying devices to deliver the correct amount of radiation to the tumor while sparing the maximum amount of normal tissue. Oftentimes, several plans are attempted by the dosimetrist and oncologist before the best plan is selected. Finally, another type of radiation specialist called a medical physicist, verifies that both the radiation treatment plan and the actual treatment machines are precise and free from errors using a variety of rigorous quality assurance tests. Physicists test the software and hardware of all the computers and radiation machines throughout the entire process. After the plan is completed and checked many times by physicians, dosimetrists, and physicists, the patient is scheduled for their first treatment.

At the beginning of each treatment, a radiation therapist (RTT) accompanies the patient into the treatment room and aligns them in the proper position on the treatment table. The RTT is responsible for verifying an accurate setup and delivering the radiation treatment each day. The initial treatment may take a little longer than the subsequent treatments because extra imaging and measurements are taken to confirm a proper setup. Throughout the course of treatment, verification films and other checks are regularly performed to confirm accuracy in patient setup and radiation delivery. While under treatment, radiation team members, including RTTs, physicians, physician assistants, nurse practitioners, and nurses will see each patient and address questions or issues that may occur. Remember, X-ray treatment does not hurt. In fact, the most common complaints that I hear from patients during treatments are how far patients must drive to get to the cancer center and how hard the table is that they must lie on. Nevertheless, as treatments progress, fatigue and other side effects become more of a factor to many patients.

Radiation not only kills or slows the growth of cancer cells; it can also affect nearby healthy cells. Damage to healthy cells can cause side effects. Side effects that appear during or shortly after radiation are called acute side effects. They are usually temporary and generally diminish over time after treatment is completed. Radiation therapy side effects depend on which part of your body is being exposed to radiation and how much radiation is used. You may experience no side effects, or you may experience several. One of the most common side effects is fatigue—a feeling of exhaustion that may start quickly or come on slowly. Like many other symptoms, people feel fatigue in different ways, and you may feel more fatigue or less fatigue than someone else who is getting the same amount of radiation therapy to the same part of the body. Please refer to Table 2 to see a list of common side effects with X-ray treatments. Discuss this chart with your doctor or nurse. Ask them about your chances of experiencing each side effect.

Table 2. Possible Side Effects from Radiation (X-ray) Therapy

Brain

- Fatigue
- Hair loss (treatment area only)
- Nausea and vomiting
- Skin changes/redness (treatment area only)
- Headache
- Blurry vision

Breast

- Fatigue
- Hair loss (treatment area only)
- Skin changes/redness (treatment area only)
- Swelling (Edema)
- Tenderness

Chest

- Fatigue
- Hair loss (treatment area only)
- Skin changes/redness (treatment area only)
- Throat changes, such as trouble swallowing
- Cough
- Shortness of breath

Head and Neck

- Fatigue
- Hair loss (treatment area only)
- Mouth changes (dry mouth-possibly permanent)
- Skin changes/redness (treatment area only)
- Taste changes
- Throat changes, such as trouble swallowing
- Less active thyroid gland

Pelvis

- Diarrhea
- Fatigue
- Hair loss (treatment area only)
- Nausea and vomiting
- Sexual problems (men)
- Fertility problems (men)
- Sexual problems (women)
- Fertility problems (women)
- Skin changes/redness (treatment area only)
- Urinary and bladder changes

Rectum

- Diarrhea
- Fatigue
- Hair loss (treatment area only)
- Sexual problems (men)
- Fertility problems (men)
- Sexual problems (women)
- Fertility problems (women)
- Skin changes/redness (treatment area only)
- Urinary and bladder changes

Stomach and Abdomen

- Diarrhea
- Fatigue
- Hair loss (treatment area only)
- Nausea and vomiting
- Skin changes/redness (treatment area only)
- Urinary and bladder changes

Website: National Cancer Institute, May 1, 2018; https://www.cancer.gov/about-cancer/treatment/types/radiation-therapy/side-effects

Healthy cells that are damaged during radiation treatment usually recover in the weeks to months after treatment is over. Sometimes, however, people may have side effects that do not improve. Other side effects may show up months or years after radiation therapy is over. These are called late effects and are more likely to be permanent or long-lasting. The likelihood of developing late side effects depends on the part of your body that was treated, other types of previous treatments, genetics, lifestyle choices (i.e. smoking), and other factors. Late side effects that occur within the treatment area may sometimes include heart issues, lung scarring, dry mouth, swelling of the extremity, skin darkening, and even secondary cancers from treatment. Ask your doctor or nurse which late effects you should watch for. See the section on Late Effects (https://www.cancer.gov/about-cancer/coping/survivorship/late-effects) to learn more.

One of the most feared late side effects deserves special mention—Radiation-Induced Secondary Malignancy (RISM), also known as a secondary cancer. While there is a real risk of radiation therapy causing secondary cancers, I believe that its impact on decision-making is greatly exaggerated. A disproportionate fear associated with radiation treatments has caused some patients to ignore the immediate threat and much greater chance of dying of the cancer that is staring them in the face. In a practical sense, a small chance of a treatment-induced malignancy should not prevent a patient from receiving treatment for a serious cancer. It helps to realize that radiation-induced cancers are relatively uncommon and usually less of a factor than other genetic factors or lifestyle choices. Four major areas are known to impact secondary cancer risks – 1) age, 2) genetics, 3) tissue/organ treatment site, and 4) volume of irradiated tissue[1]. To label a cancer as a RISM, it is important to recognize that it must occur within the radiation treatment field and usually requires five to twenty years after radiation to develop. Some argue that the risk is lower with modern treatments since treatment areas are often smaller and radiation doses are less than older treatment regimens.

The Childhood Cancer Survivors Study group analyzed over 14,000 survivors of pediatric malignancies and found that 7.9% of all these patients developed a secondary cancer at 30 years after their original primary cancer diagnosis. The total number of secondary malignancies was higher among those who received radiation (10%) versus those who did not (5%). Therefore, radiation exposure seems to increase the risk of secondary cancers in children by about 5%. They also report that radiation exposure impacts children significantly more than older populations. The risk is higher in children because they are more susceptible to treatment and have more time for a tumor to develop during their lifetime. For a given dose, children are around tenfold more sensitive to develop RISM as compared to adults[2,3]. Despite multiple confounding factors, I think for adults it is reasonable to estimate the risk of a secondary cancer to be less than 1% overall. For a more complete list of side effects from cancer treatments in general, please visit the National Cancer Institute (NCI) website at: https://www.cancer.gov/about-cancer/treatment/side-effects.

CHAPTER SEVEN

WHAT ELSE SHOULD I CONSIDER WHEN CHOOSING TREATMENT?

When faced with cancer it is difficult to know where to turn. After a biopsy, medical scans, and cancer staging, it is time to consider treatment options.

Do your homework and go with your gut. Turn to trusted friends and family. Use both local and national resources. Don't be afraid to learn about your diagnosis from sources like the internet but be wary; not everything you read will be true. Your focus needs to be finding the right team to help you decide on the right treatment for you.

WHERE SHOULD I SEEK TREATMENT?

It is true that some of the greatest oncologists in the world work at large academic institutions like those of the NCCN, but there are also great doctors who fight cancer every day in smaller cancer centers around the country. So, when should you accept treatment from a local cancer center and when should you uproot your life for a few months to travel to a faraway cancer center? In my opinion, it depends on where you live and what type of cancer you have. That decision is very specific and occasionally even I have difficulty knowing which doctors to choose unless it is an area with which I am very familiar. Most people are pleased with the care they receive from their local cancer center, but occasionally, it is better to seek treatment far from home.

An advantage of a local cancer center is that it is local. You can continue much of your regular life without interruption. Some people can work throughout their entire cancer treatment, but this really depends on the type of cancer and treatment. You should not try to "tough it out" when you are sick. With some treatments it is simply not possible to maintain your normal activities or work schedule. Sometimes just getting out of bed or eating a meal is a success. It really depends on your situation and I encourage you to discuss what to expect and how you are doing with your healthcare team. Seeking treatment locally also causes less disruption to your loved ones. It may allow you to continue participating in family events or activities that would be missed during out-of-state travel. Not only are you surrounded by people and things you love, but it is also considerably cheaper to stay at home. Hotels, gas, and airline tickets can add up quickly. If a surgery you need is rare or extensive, you might consider finding a surgeon with a lot of experience performing that surgery. On the other hand, most surgeries, chemotherapies, and radiation treatments are going to be very similar regardless of where you seek treatment. Large, academic medical centers will work with local cancer doctors to create a treatment regimen right for you.

SHOULD I GET A SECOND OPINION?

The main reason people travel is to seek advice and sometimes treatment from the best or most experienced cancer centers. Sometimes this is unnecessary, particularly for standard treatment, but occasionally it makes a big difference. While a local oncologist has likely treated each of the common types of cancer hundreds of times, large cancer centers have teams of doctors that sub-specialize in every possible type of cancer. As a general radiation oncologist, I treat cancers head-to-toe in children and adults. A typical day may include breast, prostate, lung, brain, H&N, GI, and GYN cancers. At a large academic center, you may see a specialist that only treats one type of cancer and knows everything there is to know about his/her area of expertise. However, this knowledge may or may not translate into a better treatment for you. If it is a common cancer, probably not. If it is a rare or recurrent cancer or there is something unusual about your case, it might be worth the trip. Many people seek a consultation with a world expert to get the best game plan and then arrange for treatment to be delivered at a local cancer center. It is common for oncologists at major cancer centers to spell out a plan on paper and coordinate care with local physicians. Oncologists work in teams, so it is normal to accept input from other centers—this is done every day. By the way, my rule of thumb regarding second opinions is that if your local doctor knows what he/she is talking about then they won't mind you getting a second opinion. They might even encourage it because it only proves they were right all along. On the other hand, if a doctor advises you not to get a second opinion, you might want to run and get one!

WHAT ABOUT RESEARCH TRIALS?

While it is truly amazing how far medical research and technology have advanced in the last few decades, there will always be more questions to answer. With new medicines and treatments, oncologists must ask the same basic questions all over again in regard to the new treatments. Is the new medicine better than the last? If so, how much is best? Should the new treatment be given before, during, or after another successful treatment? This constant questioning of new therapies goes on and on. The results of cancer research take at least five to ten years to form preliminary answers to many of these types of questions. Oncologists may offer you the opportunity to participate in research trials that are actively enrolling patients to help find the answers. If you are not interested in participating or not eligible for research trials, don't worry; you will still be offered the best available treatments based on the current level of medical knowledge and accepted standards of care.

There are ongoing cancer research trials from various medical centers around the world. Many cancer centers participate in research studies designed by teams of oncology experts who joined together to form cooperative research groups like the National Cancer Institute (NCI), NRG Oncology (joint organization of the NSABP, RTOG, and GOG), European Organization for Research and Treatment of Cancer (EORTC), and many others. A group of the top-tier cancer centers in the U.S. joined to form the National Comprehensive Cancer Network (NCCN). The NCCN publishes guidelines that act like a "cookbook" for oncologists around the world. Some of our best treatments come from the results of these research groups. The trials of today represent the cutting-edge of where we are in the fight against cancer. Participation should always be encouraged if the situation fits and if the patient is eligible for a trial. While there is usually no financial incentive, patients still benefit by receiving the best care available. To be fair, there is some level of uncertainty about the experimental arm of a research trial (that is why the trial exists), but the treatments have been evaluated by boards of researchers and physicians to confirm that the new treatments have a meaningful and rational chance to improve treatment results while being as safe as possible. Perhaps an even greater benefit is the personal satisfaction of knowing that you are contributing to the body of knowledge that may help others in the future.

CAN STATISTICS HELP ME CHOOSE THE RIGHT TREATMENT?

When diagnosed with cancer, one is confronted with their own mortality and thrust into unfamiliar situations in a hospital or doctor's office. Throughout this journey, it helps to be reminded that when we are deciding how to treat your body—you're the boss. I don't care what somebody in a white coat tells you, he/she does not have to live with the consequences of your decision. Don't misunderstand me; your doctor deserves respect, should be listened to, and is generally going to be right about most cancer issues, but you're still in charge. Ask questions and bring a friend to listen or take notes at your initial consultations. Ultimately, no one can do something for you (or to you) that you don't want. If you haven't already done so, it would benefit you to appoint a medical power of attorney and complete a living will to educate your family about your wishes. When making treatment decisions don't forget to try to weigh the benefits versus the risks of each treatment option. More is not always better—sometimes it is just more. Ask the physician what he would do if you were his/her family member. You might also consider asking questions like:

> Why do you recommend treatment?
> What is my chance of a permanent cure?
> What are the odds of me living longer?
> What will my quality of life be like?
> How long should the temporary side effects last?
> What kind of permanent side effects does this treatment cause?

Doctors must interpret tremendous amounts of information, but we are not always great at predicting how long individual patients may live. We can estimate how long an "average" patient survives with a cancer, but that doesn't always translate in a meaningful way to the individual sitting in front of you. This can be illustrated by a high school math test. The class average on a final exam may be a "B", but one student received an "A+" and another student failed—same goes for cancer. For example, if a cancer has a cure rate of 70% (7 out of 10) that does not mean that the person sitting in the doctor's office is in the 70%. He or she could be in the 30% (3 out of 10) that is not cured. It's difficult to know for sure until the patient has been around for a few years.

Some knowledge of statistics may also be helpful for patients. In statistics, a mathematically significant result doesn't always translate into real world significance. For example, randomized data in women with breast cancer who are treated with a lumpectomy and are older than 70 years of age with very favorable breast cancers (stage T1N0M0 with small tumors, no spread to lymph nodes, negative surgical margins, positive estrogen receptors (ER+), and who agree to take anastrozole for 5 years) show that radiation therapy statistically decreases cancer recurrences from about 10% to less than 2%[1]. Is this significant in the real world? To some it may be, but both groups have better than a 9 out of 10 chance that their cancer won't ever come back. Surgery and hormone therapy cured at least 90% and adding 3 weeks of radiation treatment bumped up the local control to 98%. Which would you choose? Would it change your mind to know that the overall survival of both groups of patients was the same? It cannot be proven that adding radiation to this particular group of patients would make anybody live longer. How can this be if the local recurrence rate dropped from 10% to 2%? Shouldn't at least 8% (8 out of 100) of women live longer? Not necessarily, because almost all those women will either die of diseases other than cancer or if it does come back, they will likely be cured by additional surgery, like a mastectomy. Please don't misunderstand, this applies only to this situation. If these older women had larger tumors or spread to the lymph nodes, it is an entirely different situation. Outside of this specific exception discussed above, radiation following lumpectomy has been shown to decrease recurrence, increase cure, and help women live longer. The details are important so be sure to discuss them with your doctor and find out as much as possible before making treatment decisions.

Some statistics that are helpful in guiding oncologists are median survival and overall survival. *Median survival* is the length of time that half the people died, and half are still alive. By definition, half the people live more than whatever number the doctor says, and half the people live less. It still surprises me how many patients misunderstand this statistic. If a doctor says that the median survival is 6 months—it does NOT mean that you have 6 months to live. It means that half the people didn't make it to 6 months and the other half lived more than 6 months. I sometimes find it helpful to look at the range of survival as well. Some of those same people may be alive many years later, while others might not have survived through treatment. Another statistic, *overall survival,* equals the percentage of people that are alive at a certain point in time— usually 1, 2, 5, or 10 years down the road. It is generally assumed that if you're alive and cancer free at 10 years or so, there is a good chance that specific cancer is not coming back. Why? Because it would've come back already. Fast-growing cancers, like some lymphomas, lung cancer, cervix cancer, and squamous cell carcinomas of the head & neck, usually come back in the first couple of years if they are ever going to come back. There are always exceptions, but generally speaking, if microscopic remnants of these faster cancers are hiding somewhere in the body, they will usually grow big enough to be seen on a scan or to cause a symptom within the first 2–3 years, and even more likely by 5 years after treatment. Prostate cancer, breast cancer, and some other "slower" cancers, can come back even 15 years later. Also, it helps to recognize that many oncologists don't ever use the word cure. I don't think that's fair to the patient because most people that haven't had their cancer come back after 5–10 years really are cured for life. That does NOT mean, however, that they couldn't develop a totally different and unrelated cancer. If you are breathing, you can develop a cancer—it is a risk of being alive.

Furthermore, I do not believe that we are all walking around with cancer waiting to spread. I've heard patients remark that we all have cancer in our body, but that is not accurate. We simply cannot know if or when a person's cells will undergo the right mutations to push a normal cell into becoming a cancer cell. There are many biochemical steps which must happen for this to occur, but that is beyond the scope of this text. There are also many other measures that oncologists track and consider, such as local or regional control, rate of distant metastasis, disease-free survival, and cancer-specific survival. To understand how oncologists use statistics, let's look closer at disease-free survival.

Disease-free survival (DFS) is the percentage of patients that are alive AND without evidence of disease at some point in time after treatment. Please understand that the 5-year overall survival is how many people are alive 5 years later, but 5-year DFS is how many people are alive AND do not have any detectable disease on their physical examination and medical imaging (i.e. CT, MRI or PET scans). To highlight the difference, consider two cancers with relatively high cure rates—Hodgkin's lymphoma and prostate cancer. Hodgkin's disease is generally seen in young people (teens-thirties) while prostate cancer is typically seen in older men. While *overall survival* is important in both, DFS is more helpful in prostate cancer decision-making than in Hodgkin's lymphoma patients. Why? To understand, consider how many years of life remain for each group of patients. Teenagers with Hodgkin's disease are expected to live for many decades if cured and there are few other life-threatening illnesses that typically occur in the short-term. Men over 60 with prostate cancer are on the downhill side of life and have a much higher chance of dying of heart attack, stroke, or some other disease associated with aging. The reason DFS is important is that the goal of these statistical endpoints is to determine if a treatment is effective and worthwhile. DFS and overall survival are likely to be very similar in the young patient with Hodgkin's lymphoma because cancer is the biggest threat to survival. Young people usually don't die of heart attacks. On the other hand, overall survival in older patients is obscured by competing causes of death so DFS tells us more about the effectiveness of a cancer treatment. Ten years after both of these groups were treated, the older men dying of heart attacks may have been cured of prostate cancer; however, the results of our treatment are hidden by other unrelated problems; this is one of the problems we face in oncology statistics.

You might be thinking that if the prostate cancer patient was going to die of a heart attack anyway, then "who cares about prostate cancer?" Well, you might care if you were a relatively healthy 60-year-old that goes to the gym 3 times per week, eats right, and has a family history of men living into their 90's. Suddenly, the threat of prostate cancer becomes the most likely thing to take you out over the next 25 years. Maybe we should also look at something other than just overall survival, hence the use of DFS. There are many other statistics to measure and it can become an area of confusion. A reason why a doctor may give a differing opinion about which treatment is best for a patient is that he sometimes places different weight on different cancer statistics. Furthermore, measuring *quality* of life is even more difficult because people possess different sets of values and rate symptoms differently. Ultimately, the patient should decide which treatment option is best for them. Please discuss these statistics with your oncologist or health care team to understand these terms better and clarify which treatment regimens may be best for you.

WHAT ABOUT ALTERNATIVE THERAPIES AND NUTRITION?

The American Society of Clinical Oncology (ASCO) released the second annual National Cancer Opinion Survey in October 2018[1] that revealed:

"Nearly four in 10 Americans believe cancer can be cured solely through alternative therapies (like diet modification), despite evidence that patients who use alternative therapies instead of standard cancer treatments have much higher mortality rates."

This survey included nearly 5,000 U.S. adults, with over 1,000 participants having already had a cancer. While there are several interesting findings, one concern is the very high percentage of patients that falsely believe that alternative therapies are as effective as standard medical treatments for cancer. Unfortunately, there is good evidence that this claim is false. The survival rates of cancer patients that choose only alternative therapies over currently accepted cancer treatment regimens have only about half the likelihood of surviving their cancer. Another study[2] identified 281 patients with non-metastatic breast, prostate, lung, or colorectal cancer who chose alternative medicines as their sole anticancer treatment rather than conventional cancer treatments defined as chemotherapy, radiotherapy, surgery, and/or hormone therapy. The patients who solely used alternative medicines had a 2.5 times greater risk of death compared with conventional cancer treatments while in subgroups with breast, lung, and colorectal cancer the risk of death was 5.7, 2.2, and 4.6 times greater in patients choosing alternative treatments, respectively. While some alternative therapies may complement traditional medical treatments, some may do more harm than good. I recommend you discuss any alternative treatments openly with your oncologist and other physicians.

Nevertheless, it cannot be overstated that nutrition is critically important during and after cancer treatments. Plenty of fluids are important for the proper functioning of the heart, kidneys and many other organs. Fiber is important to maintain regular bowel movements and gastrointestinal function. Protein is very important to give your body the building blocks and raw materials to be able to repair itself from treatments like surgery, chemotherapy, and radiation. Since radiation works by creating free radicals inside tumor cells, large doses of antioxidants are not generally recommended during radiation therapy, although a daily multivitamin is generally acceptable. It is critical that one does not diet or restrict food consumption during or shortly after cancer treatments because the body is already stressed and needs nourishment. Many patients misunderstand the role of eating sugar during cancer treatment. While it is true that cancers also use sugar, it is important to remember that a tumor will get whatever nutrients it wants from your body whether you eat sugar or not. Tumors, like a baby during pregnancy, get preferential treatment from the body. By depriving yourself of sugar, you are also likely limiting other important nutrients from food that you desperately need. Good evidence exists that patients who lose more than 5% of their body weight suffer a worse prognosis than those who do not[3]. Other lifestyle recommendations that will help you to recover more quickly are to avoid alcohol and tobacco, exercise lightly, and get plenty of sleep.

CHAPTER EIGHT

WHAT HAPPENS AFTER TREATMENTS ARE FINISHED?

R egardless of whatever treatment regimen is given, at some point it will be completed. After treatment, patients can expect to see gradual improvement in acute side effects for several weeks. Your doctor(s) will usually schedule a series of follow-up appointments (about every 1–3 months) that are gradually spaced out to be less frequent as time goes by. Lab tests or medical scans may be ordered before follow-up appointments to assess whether the cancer has responded to treatment or not. These tests are used to see if the cancer is in remission, or if it has grown or spread. If there is no evidence of cancer, routine follow-up appointments will continue as scheduled. If the cancer returns, called a recurrence, your oncologist may order additional tests to "re-stage" the cancer. Once the new extent of disease is determined, a new treatment plan will be developed and discussed with you. Some salvage cancer treatments are very successful while others are not. Treatment for recurrences sometimes have different or more serious side effects than the initial cancer treatment, but this depends on the specifics of each case. Just like the first time, it is important to ask questions and try to understand as much as possible about your treatment options. As always, the ultimate decision of how to proceed is up to you.

WHAT IS THE ROLE OF PALLIATIVE CARE AND HOSPICE?

To claim that a cancer is not curable means that no further treatment options have a reasonable chance of killing all the tumor cells in the body. It does not mean that a patient is not treatable. When cure is not possible, treatments may still prolong life or increase quality of life by preventing serious symptoms. The goal of these treatments is considered palliative rather than curative. Some palliative treatments help patients live longer. Others help relieve pain, bleeding, bowel obstruction, and other types of suffering. Palliative cancer treatments may include chemotherapy, hormonal therapy, radiation therapy, and other treatments. About half of the patients that I see in my radiation oncology practice were treated with the goal of cure, while the other half came for palliation of symptoms. Even if a patient enrolls in hospice or comfort measures, there may still be a role for palliative cancer treatments. For example, one of the roles of radiation therapy is to relieve severe pain. Radiation treatment is highly effective in relieving bone pain and pressure from tumors that push on nerves and other tissues. About 3 out of 4 patients experience significant pain relief from a short course of these X-ray treatments, sometimes in even one treatment.

While some believe that narcotics alone are enough to provide pain relief at the end stages of life, this is not always best. To relieve cancer pain, some patients require such high levels of narcotics that they are essentially unconscious. Families must watch their loved one be either awake and in pain or asleep. Palliative therapy may provide a quick and easy way to decrease the severity of pain and subsequent demand for narcotics so that patients can be conscious and enjoy time with their family or have meaningful end-of-life conversations. Unfortunately, many patients, providers, and care facilities are not aware of this important role of radiation treatments. Thankfully, there is a recent trend to use multidisciplinary teams to guide patients through end-of-life care. Another little-known fact is that patients can voluntarily resign from hospice programs in order to receive a palliative treatment and then re-enlist in hospice to take full advantage of all available comfort measures.

In my opinion, hospice services are one of the most underutilized services in healthcare. Most people wait until the last few days of life and miss out on months of benefit from some of the most caring people in all of medicine. Please don't be afraid to ask about comfort care programs. There are no right and wrong choices in deciding how you choose to face these life and death decisions. It is important to realize that your medical team will continue to care for you even if you decide to discontinue active cancer therapies. Palliative care teams and hospice workers support patients through end-of-life care and emphasize their quality of life.

PART TWO

SPECIFIC TYPES OF CANCER

For the remainder of this book, each chapter will focus on a specific type of cancer. While all patients can benefit from the general principals in Part I, it is not necessary to read all of Part II. I recommend you skip to the chapter on the type of cancer that you're interested in learning about. I've attempted to organize each chapter by symptoms, workup, pathology, treatment, and other unique features surrounding that type of cancer. My goal is to highlight major topics and issues I think will best help you. It is important that you find an oncologist you are comfortable with and that you trust. There are many other types of cancer that we will not specifically cover, including less common situations, like childhood cancers, but hopefully this short booklet will help you sort through the most common issues. The following chapters include cancers of the brain, breast, gastrointestinal (GI) tract, gynecologic (GYN) organs, head & neck, lung, lymph nodes/bone marrow, prostate, and skin. For additional information regarding other cancer questions, I *highly recommend* the websites of the **American Cancer Society** at http://www.cancer.org and the **National Cancer Institute (NCI)** at https://www.cancer.gov or you can contact me directly at http://www.AskTheCancerDoc.com.

CHAPTER ONE

BRAIN TUMORS

Brain tumors come in two varieties: 1) **Brain metastasis**—cancers that spread from somewhere else in the body and 2) **Primary brain tumors** that originate from tissues within the brain (*gliomas, meningiomas, pituitary adenomas*). Both types of brain tumors may cause symptoms, such as headache, nausea, vomiting, seizures, visual loss, hearing loss, nerve damage, paralysis, or other serious neurologic problems depending on which part of the brain is affected. Some of these symptoms simply result from direct pressure of the tumor or from swelling (edema) around the tumor that pushes on the brain. This pressure on the brain, called increased intracranial pressure, is usually the first cause of symptoms, particularly headaches and nausea. Fortunately, a steroid medicine called dexamethasone can be used to relieve these symptoms. Dexamethasone is fast and effective at controlling most brain symptoms, but may result in other side effects such as increased appetite, elevated blood sugar, nervousness, insomnia, swelling of the face or extremities, gradual loss of strength in the thigh muscles of the legs, etc. Most of these medicine-induced side effects are just a nuisance and a small price to pay to control the life-threatening effects of increased brain pressure caused by tumors in the brain.

Workup of brain tumor symptoms usually involves a CT scan of the head and an MRI of the brain with intravenous (IV) contrast. CT scan shows the bones, sinuses, and soft tissues of the head very well, but MRI of the brain is far better at imaging the brain itself. Typically, if a patient presents with a new and rapid onset of headache, a CT of the head is first performed to rule out an emergent and hemorrhagic (bleeding) stroke. Otherwise, an MRI of the brain will be ordered to investigate the fine details of the brain tissue and blood vessels within the brain. MRI is used to identify strokes, tumors, infection, swelling (edema), or other brain abnormalities. If a mass or tumor is seen, then a neurosurgeon is usually consulted to consider performing a biopsy. As we discussed in Part I of this book, a tissue diagnosis via pathologic review of a biopsy specimen is the only way to know for sure what type of cancer we are dealing with on a scan. Sometimes, a brain biopsy or resection is the first step in a patient's cancer journey. Other times, a new brain mass on an MRI scan can be reasonably assumed to be a metastasis from a patient's previously known cancer and a biopsy is not necessary.

The most common origin of brain tumors is from a cancer that started somewhere else in the body, particularly cancer of the lung, breast, colon, renal cell carcinoma of the kidney, or melanoma cancer of the skin. While brain metastasis can occur from any cancer, the five types that I mention here represent the most common culprits for producing cancer cells that spread through the blood and grow in the brain. These tumor metastases to the brain are considered Stage IV and are generally not curable. The rare exception to this rule is tumors that are extremely sensitive to chemotherapy—like classic testicular seminomas. In general, prognosis for patients with brain metastasis is not good, but treatment is slowly getting better. For a single brain metastasis, traditional treatment was surgical resection followed by ten daily radiation treatments to the whole brain over 2 weeks. Whole-brain radiation treats the tumors that can be seen on MRI and CT scans, but also treats the microscopic tumor cells that we must assume are hiding in the brain that are too small to be seen on medical imaging. The downside to treating the whole brain is the increase in side effects, particularly neurocognitive changes such as memory loss, confusion, and hypersomnolence (excessive sleepiness). Other side effects of whole-brain treatment include hair loss, fatigue, scalp redness, nausea, headache, endocrine abnormalities, and other symptoms.

Recent advances in treating brain metastasis allow radiation treatment to just the brain lesions themselves, as opposed to treating the whole brain. Sophisticated radiation treatments that target only the tumor, called focal radiation, can deliver very high doses of radiation with amazing accuracy and precision without treating the surrounding normal tissues of the brain. They include stereotactic radiosurgery (SRS)—in one treatment, or stereotactic body radiation therapy (SBRT)—in two to five treatments. Today, many patients receive SRS or SBRT for single or multiple brain metastasis with better results. The higher doses focused only on the tumor results in local tumor control of better than 90%. In other words, focal stereotactic radiation allows more than 9 out of 10 of these metastases to be killed with fewer side effects, and much less impact on neurocognitive (brain) function. The only drawback of treating just the brain tumor is that the remaining "good" brain is left untreated and there is a higher risk that unseen tumors may grow there in the future. Fortunately, focal stereotactic radiation may be repeated, if necessary, to new areas and sometimes even to the same area that was already treated. By the way, it is also important to point out that for multiple brain metastasis, radiation therapy is preferred over brain surgery (craniotomy) because surgery adds to the side effects without improving overall survival. Nevertheless, craniotomy to surgically remove all or part of a tumor is sometimes warranted to obtain a diagnosis of cancer or to rapidly relieve symptoms of pressure from larger lesions that push on the brain.

The second variety of brain tumors that we must recognize arise from normal brain cells that undergo mutations to transform into cancer cells, however, they do NOT tend to spread to other parts of the body. These types of brain tumors, called primary brain tumors, may be considered benign or malignant. Benign brain tumors usually grow very slowly and are not usually lethal but can still push on nerves and cause problems to nearby tissues. These benign tumors may require surgery and/or focal radiation therapy and include meningiomas, schwannomas, pituitary adenomas, and the like. Malignant brain tumors are more aggressive, grow more quickly, and are often deadly. While there are many types of malignant brain tumors, the most common type is a class of brain tumor called gliomas. Gliomas are categorized by a special grading system designed by the World Health Organization, aptly called the WHO grading system. The WHO system ranks glioma brain tumors from least to most aggressive (grade I—*pilocytic astrocytoma*, grade II—*low grade gliomas*, grade III—*anaplastic astrocytomas*, and grade IV— *glioblastomas*). The prognosis of these malignant gliomas varies by grade, size, age of the patient, performance status, and a host of other factors. Treatment of low-grade gliomas (WHO grade I & II) is often surgical resection alone, but high-grade gliomas (WHO III & IV) are best treated with surgical resection, radiation therapy, and often chemotherapy. A multidisciplinary approach involving neurosurgeons, radiation oncologists, and medical oncologists are required to achieve the best results.

Glioblastomas (WHO grade IV) require a biopsy for diagnosis and complete surgical resection is recommended if possible. Many times, these tumors cannot be safely resected because they infiltrate critical areas of the brain and resections would cause unacceptable complications like death, paralysis, or permanent disability. A few weeks after surgery, patients are referred for radiation therapy to maximize the chances of killing as much tumor as possible, while preventing symptoms and prolonging life. Prior to starting treatment, the radiation therapy team will create a plastic customized facemask for radiation treatment planning. The mask fits tightly so the patient's head is immobilized during treatment. After the mask is created, a CT scan (called a CT simulation or CT sim) is done at the same appointment that usually lasts a total of about 30 minutes. After the appointment, the CT images are transferred digitally to a specialized treatment planning computer where the radiation team generates a radiation plan. Radiation oncologists, medical dosimetrists, and medical physicists create, analyze, and verify the accuracy of a radiation treatment plan. The quality assurance process that must be completed prior to radiation planning and delivery is extensive and is of the utmost importance. Only after passing multiple evaluations is the plan deemed ready for treatment and the patient called to return for the start of treatment. Traditionally, treatment for gliomas requires about 30 treatments that each take about 15 minutes per day, given 5 days per week for a total of 6 weeks. For some patients, recent research shows that shorter radiation treatment regimens (hypofractionation) may be given via fewer fractions over shorter periods of time. Glioblastoma patients also respond better if a chemotherapy pill, temozolomide, is given daily during and after radiation therapy. A new form of therapy for these aggressive brain tumors following standard surgery and chemoradiation, known as Tumor-Treating Field therapy (Optune™), delivers electric fields to disrupt mitosis and tumor growth. This treatment involves placing adhesive pads directly onto the scalp for several hours each day and has been shown in some studies to improve overall survival. Unfortunately, the statistics show that most glioblastomas recur later in the same part of the brain as they began so be sure to follow-up with your scans and appointments.

After radiation treatment for either brain metastasis or primary brain tumors, follow-up MRI scans of the brain may be ordered every few months to assess whether the treatment area is stable (the tumor isn't growing) and that there are no new tumors. High-dose, focal radiation treatments may kill all the tumor cells at the treatment area but often cause a scar that can be seen on MRI scans. Radiation (X-ray) treatment sometimes irritates or damages the normal tissues in the treatment area, called radiation necrosis, and may result in symptoms that imitate tumor recurrence. Radiation necrosis may also mimic the appearance of recurrent tumor on MRI scans and cause anxiety for patients. Treatment for necrosis *and* tumor recurrence includes dexamethasone, close follow up with MRI scans, and occasionally surgery. Sometimes, another medicine called bevacizumab may be used to decrease swelling or leakage from blood vessels that cause necrosis. Be sure to discuss the details of all the available treatment options with your doctor.

Family and friends often play a significant role in facing the many challenges of dealing with tumors of the brain. If you have questions or concerns at any time, do not hesitate to contact your oncologist or family doctor. For more on chemotherapy and/or radiation side effects from treatment, please refer to Tables 1 & 2 of Chapter 6 in Part I of this book. For additional information regarding other cancer questions, please visit the websites mentioned in the Foreword.

CHAPTER TWO

BREAST CANCER

Breast cancer is the most common cancer in American women (lifetime risk is 1 out of 8 women) and occasionally even occurs in men. Yet, a diagnosis of breast cancer can strike fear in the heart. Much has been written about breast cancer and, in many ways, has been a flagship cancer to raise awareness about all other cancers. There are many important tumor factors that help doctors estimate the aggressiveness of breast cancers. It is overwhelming for a patient to consider all the issues that guide modern treatment recommendations for breast cancer. Some of the prognostic factors include tumor size, location, number of involved lymph nodes, tumor grade, estrogen/progesterone/Her-2 neu status, patient age, and specific genetic markers that oncologists are just starting to understand. Let's explore some breast cancer basics.

The purpose of the breast is to produce milk for lactation. For reasons that we don't understand, most breast cancers begin in the cells of the milk ducts. If these cells undergo mutations and turn cancerous, they most often become a type of cancer known as an adenocarcinoma. Adenocarcinomas of the milk ducts are known, not surprisingly as ductal carcinomas. If they are non-invasive (i.e. stay within the milk ducts), they are called **ductal carcinoma in-situ (DCIS)** because "in-situ" means "in place". If they invade through the wall of the milk duct, they are called **invasive ductal carcinomas**. Invasive ductal carcinomas are taken more seriously than DCIS because after they invade through the duct, they can then spread to lymph nodes or other parts of the body. Breast cancers are usually discovered by a routine screening mammogram or they are palpated (felt with the fingers) by the patient or her (his) doctor. It is not unusual for mammograms to miss small tumors that are palpable. It is also common to see tumors on mammograms that cannot be palpated. Today, higher definition three-dimensional (3D) breast tomography and ultrasound are helping to detect smaller breast lesions than ever before, but no test is perfect. Even a breast MRI has the problem of confusing benign tissues with "would-be tumors", which pushes the patient into unnecessary biopsies and should therefore be limited to specific instances.

If a suspicious area is detected, the next step is a core needle biopsy to confirm a diagnosis of cancer. If the biopsy is positive, additional medical scans may be ordered, and an oncologic surgery is needed. An oncologic surgery is a type of surgery to completely remove (cut out) a tumor or cancer while being careful not to contaminate or spread cancer cells to surrounding normal tissues by maintaining a small, continuous shell of healthy tissue around the tumor, called an en-bloc resection. Oncologic surgeries also usually include a lymph node dissection and/or sampling of any suspicious tissues at the time of surgery to see if cancer cells have spread to regional (nearby) lymph nodes. For breast cancer, an axillary lymph node dissection removes ten or more lymph nodes for both staging and treatment of the lymph node area. Recent studies have shown that a smaller surgery, called a sentinel lymph node dissection, that uses an injectable radioactive tracer or blue dye to track and remove only one to three lymph nodes is just as informative for staging purposes and has much less chance of causing permanent lymphedema, or swelling of the arm.

If the tumor is too large for a complete resection, some patients undergo chemotherapy before surgery, referred to as neoadjuvant chemotherapy, to shrink the tumor and have a better chance at removing the entire tumor. Regardless of whether chemotherapy is given or not, surgery is required. At the time of your oncologic surgery, while you are still asleep, the resected tumor specimen will be evaluated. One technique, called a specimen radiograph, uses X-rays to ensure that all the visible tumor was removed. Another technique, called an immediate frozen section, requires the tumor specimen to be sent to a pathologist who performs a rapid microscopic analysis to see if all the roots of the tumor have been removed. If all the tumor cells were not removed, the surgeon will resect more tissue during surgery until all the margins appear negative. Both the specimen radiograph and the frozen section techniques are usually accurate, but neither is infallible. It will take a couple of days after surgery for the pathologist to give a definitive answer regarding margins in a final report. This more detailed microscopic review uses a more time-consuming process to prepare the tumor specimen and analyze its cells. This official report, called a permanent section, is more accurate and worth waiting for. Occasionally, the margins are negative on frozen section and positive on permanent section and another surgery is required to take out more tissue. Based on these results, a pathologic stage can be assigned to the patient and additional treatments may be considered.

For *early-stage* breast cancer patients, the first major decision in the breast cancer journey, is also usually the most difficult. It will impact the appearance of your breast area for the rest of your life and what treatments may follow. This decision requires a choice between two surgeries. There are two basic forms of surgery to resect (cut out) breast cancer—

mastectomy and lumpectomy. Mastectomy removes the entire breast and includes variations such as a simple mastectomy (no lymph node dissection), modified radical mastectomy (includes removal of some axillary lymph nodes), and even nipple-sparing mastectomy. Lumpectomy, or breast-conserving surgery, removes a breast cancer and a small amount of surrounding normal tissue, but not the entire breast. Lumpectomy may also be referred to as a partial mastectomy, wide-local excisional biopsy, quadrantectomy, or segmental mastectomy. With the addition of other treatments, both surgeries have been scientifically proven to deliver the same rate of cure for these patients.

Cure rates for early-stage breast cancer—tumors that are small and have not spread (DCIS or T1-2 N0 M0; that is, overall stage groups 0, I, or IIA) are generally in the 90% range (9 out of 10 patients) or better. Mastectomy was the most common treatment for over a century; but today, most patients with early-stage breast cancer choose the smaller lumpectomy. Some may not require additional treatment following surgery, but most will benefit from some form of postoperative therapy. Most lumpectomy patients benefit from radiation therapy (X-ray treatment) to maximize cure following breast-conservation surgery. Many don't realize that even after a lumpectomy with negative ("good" or "clean") margins, microscopic "roots" of tumor can remain in the breast in up to 30-35% of patients. Even with the best surgeons and pathologists in the world, multiple scientific breast cancer studies have repeatedly shown that cancer cells may not all be seen under the microscope and some cells may unknowingly be missed or left behind. Please understand that these statistics mean that cancer cells following lumpectomy may remain inside the body in about one out of every three patients where the surgeon declares that they "got it all". Hidden roots of cancer, *unseen* even under a microscope, is why postoperative radiation therapy is necessary for most women with breast-conserving surgery. The good news is that radiation will "mop up" and kill any remaining cancer cells after surgery, as evidenced by the equivalent cure rates compared with the larger mastectomy.

Traditional breast radiation following lumpectomy was delivered to the entire breast area and consisted of 25-30 daily treatments over five or six weeks, but the radiation therapy options for early-stage breast cancer have improved dramatically in recent years. Today, studies have shown equivalent results with higher doses of radiation in fewer treatments, called hypo-fractionated radiation, and typically involve 15-20 daily treatments over three to four weeks to the whole breast. Another option for some early stage patients is called Partial Breast Irradiation (PBI) and treats only the area of the breast around the lumpectomy cavity rather than the entire breast. PBI may be delivered once or twice per day via ten treatments over one to two weeks using a brachytherapy device, such as a balloon catheter, or sometimes with specialized external-beam irradiation. In certain situations, PBI may even be delivered directly to the tumor margins in the operating room at the time of your oncologic surgery using a shallow form of radiation using X-rays or electron therapy. There are many unanswered questions about the best choice of technique, selection of patients for, and the overall benefit from PBI as this is still an area of active research. The main point is that radiation therapy is very effective at killing microscopic breast cancer cells that may be left behind from surgery and can be accurately delivered using a variety of modern radiation treatment techniques.

While most breast conservation patients need radiation after surgery, there are some subgroups of patients following lumpectomy with characteristics so favorable that they may *NOT* require radiation therapy. I refer to one such group as the "All-Star Team" because they have a much lower risk of recurrence than most and only require lumpectomy and hormone therapy. To be on the All-Star Team, an invasive breast cancer patient must be at least 65-70 years of age and have all the following tumor characteristics: T0-1 primary tumor (<2 cm), negative margins, no spread to lymph nodes (N0), estrogen receptor positive (ER+), and be willing to take hormone therapy for at least 5 years. For most patients that undergo lumpectomy, radiation reduces the risk of local recurrence in the breast from about 30-35% down to 5-10%, but for the All-Star Team it only decreases local recurrence from about 10% down to 1-2%[1,2]. While taking radiation therapy provides *some* improvement for this group, it is *not as much* as in most other breast cancer patients. Is it still meaningful for these postmenopausal women? Salvage mastectomy can still be done if the tumor was to recur later in the breast, so the ultimate survival of these "All-Star" patients is identical whether they decide to take radiation treatments or not. In these patients, I am comfortable deferring radiation, observing them closely, and referring them for management by a medical oncologist for hormone therapy.

Hormone therapy for breast cancer is a treatment for breast cancers that have special proteins on their cell surface, called estrogen or progesterone receptors. These hormone receptors make these cancer cells particularly sensitive to hormone therapies. The most common forms of hormone therapy for breast cancer work by blocking hormones from attaching to these receptors or by decreasing the body's production of hormones. They are sometimes used to shrink a tumor before surgery but are usually prescribed after surgery to reduce the risk that the cancer will return or help control cancer that has spread to other parts of the body. For example, it is good if your cancer is estrogen receptor positive (ER+), because medicines like tamoxifen or anastrozole modify the effects of the female hormone estrogen and help prevent cancer growth. Typically, hormone therapy is prescribed for five years, but you must discuss specific recommendations with your medical oncologist. There are some side effects, like hot flashes, endometrial bleeding, increased risk of blood clot, osteoporosis, and others that you need to consider, but these treatments have been proven to improve prognosis in the appropriate patients. Other types of receptors, such as the HER2/neu receptor, result from overexpression of oncogenes (cancer causing genes). Patients with breast cancers that are positive for the HER2/neu receptor often benefit from additional systemic therapies, such as trastuzumab or pertuzumab. There are many other receptors and details that are beyond the scope of this book and should be discussed with your medical oncologist.

We just discussed radiation and hormone treatments that sometimes follow surgery, but I want to circle back to the first decision that women must face, that of choosing between mastectomy and lumpectomy. As mentioned above, this decision not only sets the stage for which cancer treatments may follow, but also whether breast reconstruction is an option. Patients with breast-conserving surgery do not need a reconstruction, but this may be a possibility after a larger surgery. Some women choose to have only a mastectomy, while others meet with a plastic surgeon to discuss breast reconstruction. Breast reconstruction is a surgical procedure that restores shape to your breast or chest wall after a mastectomy. Breast reconstruction may be immediate (at the time of mastectomy) or delayed by several months. Reconstructions may be autologous, or "flap" reconstructions, that use a patient's own tissue, or they may involve an artificial implant filled with saline (saltwater) or silicone gel. Today, most plastic surgeons use artificial breast implants to reconstruct the breast. The implants come in a variety of sizes, shapes, and textures to fit a wide range of body types. Many reconstructions utilize an artificial balloon device that is surgically placed under the skin and slowly inflated to stretch the skin and underlying soft tissue of the chest wall. This device, aptly called a temporary tissue expander, is then replaced with the actual permanent breast implant via another surgery several months later. Breast reconstruction techniques have advanced greatly in recent years and are too extensive to fully discuss here.

While the results are much improved with modern materials and techniques, it is important to realize that a breast reconstruction will likely look and feel differently than breast augmentation or "breast implants" in women with intact breast tissue that have never undergone a mastectomy. It is common for the patient's sensation of the chest wall to be "numb" or "not have any feeling" in large areas of the skin where the breast used to be. Many women are pleased, but some are surprised or disappointed with the firm, artificial feel of the end results. Some claim that reconstruction was not worth the pain and extent of multiple surgeries; others disagree. If you are considering mastectomy, I recommend that you consult with a plastic surgeon before your oncologic surgery to learn about your options. Be sure to have the plastic surgeon show you several "before and after" pictures of his/her previous patients that underwent the same surgery that you are considering (Note: Every plastic surgeon maintains a portfolio of their outcomes so that you can see examples of their work). Also, ask for patient references with whom you can discuss what to expect. I think it best for women considering breast reconstruction to find and talk to women that have gone through this process to hear first-hand of both the good and bad experiences. Finally, remember that breast reconstruction surgery is NOT as important as the oncologic surgery to remove all the cancer cells. Reconstruction does no one any good if the cancer comes back—keep first things first.

A discussion of mastectomy and reconstruction would not be complete if I did not mention a word about bilateral (both-sided) mastectomies. Though rare, a few patients may experience bilateral breast cancer, that is, two different breast cancers—one in each breast. This unusual situation may call for an extreme treatment like bilateral mastectomies; however, most women that choose removal of both breasts do so unnecessarily out of fear. Performing a mastectomy of the "other" (contralateral) breast that does not have any evidence of cancer, called a prophylactic mastectomy, is to prevent a cancer from forming, not to treat a known cancer. Like most cancers, breast cancer can grow within the breast, spread to lymph nodes, or spread to distant parts of the body, but it usually does not spread to the other breast. I think that many women choose bilateral mastectomy because they wrongly assume that a cancer in one breast is likely to spread to the other breast, this is simply not true. The other breast does not receive a high percentage of blood flow compared to liver, lung, brain, and bones and is, therefore, less at risk. Even in rare cases where women develop a breast cancer in the other breast at the same time or later down the road, it is much more likely to be a new cancer (unrelated to the first), rather than from a cancer that spread from one breast to the other.

The irony is that women with estrogen positive cancers will likely take a hormonal pill, like anastrazole or tamoxifen, that decreases the recurrence risk in both breasts. Therefore, prophylactic or bilateral mastectomy is not necessary because the "other" (contralateral) breast in those women is *less* likely to develop a breast cancer than in women who have *never* even had a breast cancer. If we performed mastectomies for risks this low, we would have to do mastectomies on practically every woman in the country. The reason I say this is interesting is due to the shockingly high number of women who request bilateral mastectomies despite over 25 years of data that prove beyond a shadow of a doubt that lumpectomy (a smaller surgery) and radiation are just as effective as mastectomy (a larger and more difficult surgery). Since 1990, lumpectomies were being performed more regularly and it looked like mastectomies would be uncommon in early-stage breast cancer. It wasn't until the actress, Angelina Jolie, developed breast cancer and very publicly decided to undergo bilateral mastectomies that women began to request the same. Unfortunately, Angelina Jolie is one of a minority of women to be diagnosed with genetically proven breast cancer with BRCA 1 or 2 gene. This variant of breast cancer is very aggressive and is best treated with bilateral mastectomies and usually removal of the ovaries (oophorectomy) in addition to other systemic treatments. The impact of this one famous patient changed the trend away from breast conservation in the early 2000s toward these more aggressive surgeries and was a part of what became known as the 'Angelina Jolie effect'. The problem with this alarming trend is that, from an oncologic standpoint, this larger surgery is unnecessary in non-genetic breast cancer patients and often leads to excessive complications, like wound-healing problems or infections. More recent reports seem to indicate that the trend has begun to swing back toward breast-conserving therapies.

Nonetheless, for *locally advanced* breast cancers, defined as primary tumors larger than 5 cm in diameter (T3), direct invasion into the skin or muscles of the chest wall (T4), or spread to regional lymph nodes (N1, N2 or N3 cancers), radiation treatments will likely be recommended even if patients choose to have a mastectomy. Radiation following mastectomy traditionally requires 25-30 treatments over 5-6 weeks to the entire chest wall and lymph node areas, but good results from recent preliminary studies have prompted some to consider offering 15-20 hypo-fractionated treatments over 3-4 weeks. Ongoing studies will provide long-term results over the next few years that will likely confirm the safety of abbreviated hypofractionation schedules following mastectomy. It is important to point out that many women have decided to undergo the larger mastectomy instead of a breast-conserving lumpectomy in order to avoid radiation therapy altogether but were disappointed because the tumor size or lymph node involvement required radiation treatment anyway. In addition, advanced breast cancers usually require chemotherapy, regardless of the type of surgery. The decision of breast conservation surgery versus mastectomy does not affect whether the patient will need chemotherapy or not. The factors that impact the need for chemotherapy include the genetic status (Oncotype Dx score), tumor size, grade, lymph node involvement, and hormonal status; but not usually the type of surgery. If women understand that their choice of surgery may not change their need for radiation or chemotherapy, then they will be informed to make the best surgical decision for themselves. Many factors will affect your doctors' specific treatment recommendation so be sure to do your homework and ask questions about anything that doesn't make sense to you.

For women with advanced-stage breast cancer, treatment will be more extensive. Besides surgery, patients will require both chemotherapy and radiation therapy for the best results. As stated above, chemotherapy can be given before or after surgery, and the entire course usually lasts for several months. In my experience, chemotherapy is the most difficult part of treatment for most patients. If given before surgery, called neoadjuvant chemotherapy, the goal is to shrink the tumor so that it can be cut out (resected) with negative margins and possibly spare more normal tissue from being permanently removed. Neoadjuvant chemotherapy may also reduce the risk of lymphedema by decreasing tumor burden in lymph nodes and allowing less extensive axillary surgery. Finally, chemotherapy before surgery permits doctors the opportunity to assess the tumor's response to specific drugs and allow treatment to be modified accordingly. If given after surgery, the goal of chemotherapy is to kill any remaining tumor cells that might be hiding somewhere in the body. Most chemotherapy for breast cancer is usually given via an intravenous (IV) infusion directly into the bloodstream and travels all throughout the body. The most common drugs used for adjuvant and neoadjuvant chemotherapy include anthracyclines (e.g. doxorubicin), taxanes (e.g. paclitaxel, docetaxel), 5-fluorouracil (5-FU), cyclophosphamide, and carboplatin. Combinations of two or three of these drugs is often used for curative cases. For Stage IV or recurrent breast cancer, single-drug chemotherapy regimens may include these drugs, or others such as cisplatin, vinorelbine, capecitabine, gemcitabine, eribulin, or other newer agents.

One of the most common side effects of chemotherapy is extreme fatigue. I'm not talking about just needing a nap. The extreme fatigue of breast cancer chemotherapy is a "knock-your-socks-off" kind of fatigue. It has been described to me that this level of fatigue goes all the way down to your bones. The good news is that it eventually passes and there are even some patients that never experience it. Other chemotherapy side effects include a drop in white blood cells that fight infection and/or platelets that are necessary for blood to clot properly. Weekly blood draws are required to monitor these levels and adjust the chemotherapy dose accordingly. Hormonal imbalances, nausea and vomiting, hair loss, and other side effects also occur; fortunately, many of these symptoms are alleviated better than ever before with modern medicines. For nausea, pills like ondansetron, promethazine, and others, are more effective than in decades past. Intravenous (IV) forms of nausea medicine can also be given with IV fluids to "perk up" a dehydrated patient. It is a struggle, and you may lose your hair for a while, but you will make it through. Hair grows back, nausea fades—LIFE goes on.

After breast cancer treatments, follow-up examinations and scans will be done on a routine basis. Initially, you will be seen about every 3 months, but this will extend to every 6 months after a few years and eventually to an annual basis. All treatments have some side effects, and some may be permanent, but the body is resilient, and time usually helps heal most wounds. It is important to discuss any side effects, questions, or concerns with your oncologist, family doctor, and family members. For more on chemotherapy and/or radiation side effects from treatment, please refer to Tables 1 & 2 of Chapter 6 in Part I of this book. For additional information regarding other cancer questions, please visit any of the websites mentioned in the Foreword. Fighting breast cancer is difficult and life-changing, but many others have made it through, and you too can be an example for those that follow in your footsteps.

CHAPTER THREE

GASTROINTESTINAL (GI) CANCERS

The gastrointestinal (GI) tract may develop tumors that include cancers of the esophagus, stomach, pancreas, liver, colon, rectum, and anal canal. Most tumors of the GI tract are a type of cancer, called an adenocarcinoma, that usually requires surgical resection by a general surgeon. The two notable exceptions are cancers located at the upper and lower ends of the GI tract—namely esophageal and anal cancers. These two locations may develop a type of cancer, called a squamous cell carcinoma, that is generally more sensitive to the combination of chemotherapy and radiation and may not require surgical resection. Before we dive into the various treatment regimens for these various GI cancers, let's discuss some common symptoms and workup examinations for staging this class of cancers.

GI cancers may present with general symptoms like loss of appetite, early satiety, extreme fatigue, unintentional weight loss, nausea, vomiting with or without blood, abdominal pain, bloody or dark stool from digested blood, or iron deficiency anemia. The workup to evaluate these symptoms usually starts with a good history and physical and routine laboratory tests, including a CBC. The next step is often a referral to a GI doctor, called a gastroenterologist, to perform an endoscopy to identify any suspicious areas for biopsy. An endoscopy is a surgical procedure used to examine a person's digestive tract using an endoscope, a flexible tube with a light and camera that can provide color pictures and video of your digestive tract. An upper GI endoscopy is used to investigate lesions of the esophagus, stomach, pancreas, and gallbladder. A lower GI endoscopy, or colonoscopy, is used to investigate colon and rectal cancers. If a biopsy confirms the presence of cancer, the gastroenterologist may perform an additional procedure, called an endoscopic ultrasound (EUS). EUS is a minimally invasive procedure in which a special endoscope uses high-frequency sound waves (ultrasound) to visualize the depth of tumor invasion and lymph nodes for staging purposes. If a tumor is uncovered during an endoscopy examination, your oncologist will also order a CT scan of the chest, abdomen, and pelvis with IV and oral contrast (and sometimes a PET/CT) to further investigate. More recently, strange-sounding genetic biomarkers, such as MSI-H/dMMR, PD-L1, and HER2 testing, have been added to the workup of some GI tumors.

The stage and prognosis of GI cancers is based on how deep the cancer invades into the walls of the organ and the number of lymph nodes showing signs of cancer cells. Additional treatment recommendations depend on which organ is involved, the pathologic type of cancer, its stage, and the general performance status of the patient. Many of these important details are discovered from evaluating the tissue removed during an oncologic surgery and lymph node dissection. Sometimes, cancer treatments, such as chemotherapy and/or radiation therapy, may be given before (neoadjuvant), after (adjuvant), or in place of surgery. The nuances and complexity of GI cancers truly require multidisciplinary input from surgeons, medical oncologists, and radiation oncologists to achieve the best results. We will now examine some cancer treatments for the most common GI tumors.

The first organ of the GI tract, the esophagus, is a muscular tube that transports food and liquids from the mouth to the stomach. **Esophageal cancers** may cause general GI symptoms in addition to trouble swallowing, worsening indigestion or heartburn, chest pain, coughing or hoarseness. During a GI workup for esophageal cancer, a PET/CT and an endoscopy examination may reveal cancer of the upper, mid, or distal part of the esophagus or the gastro-esophageal (GE) junction and the resulting biopsy usually shows either squamous cell carcinoma or adenocarcinoma. Treatment for *early-stage* esophageal cancers (Tis, T1 N0, small T2 N0) may only require endoscopic resection or surgical removal of the esophagus, called an esophagectomy. More *advanced* esophageal cancers (T3-4, or lymph node positive—LN+) benefit from 5-6 weeks of concurrent chemotherapy and radiation (referred to as chemoradiation) either prior to a planned esophagectomy or as definitive treatment. The preferred 2-drug chemotherapy regimens may include either paclitaxel and carboplatin, fluorouracil and oxaliplatin, or fluorouracil and cisplatin. PET/CT scan may also be used after chemoradiation to assess tumor response to treatment. Tumors that respond to chemoradiation have a more favorable prognosis and may not require surgery, while patients with tumors that do not respond to treatment should undergo esophagectomy if feasible.

The second organ of the GI tract, the stomach, is a muscular organ located on the left side of the upper abdomen that receives food from the esophagus and secretes acid to digest food. Symptoms of stomach (gastric) cancer include general GI symptoms but also include stomach pain and severe, persistent indigestion, heartburn, unexplained nausea, and/or vomiting. If the endoscopy during a standard GI workup uncovers a **stomach (gastric) cancer**, the biopsy usually confirms an adenocarcinoma. An exception is a less common type of lymphoma, called a Mucosal-Associated Lymphoid Tissue (MALT) lymphoma, that is usually cured with antibiotics or radiation therapy. In contrast, treatment for *early-stage* gastric adenocarcinoma (Tis, T1 N0) may only require endoscopic resection or surgical removal of all or part of the stomach, called a gastrectomy. Likewise, more *advanced* gastric adenocarcinomas (T2-4, or lymph node positive—LN+) require surgical removal, but also benefit from fluoropyrimidine-based (fluorouracil or capecitabine) chemotherapy and/or 5-6 weeks of concurrent chemotherapy and radiation (referred to as chemo-radiation) either as preoperative, postoperative, or definitive treatment.

The next major organ of the GI tract, the pancreas, secretes enzymes and chemicals that aid in digestion. Symptoms of pancreas cancer include general GI symptoms in addition to new onset diabetes and pain in the upper abdomen that radiates to your back. Standard GI workup is further enhanced with liver function tests, a CA 19-9 blood test, and endoscopic retrograde cholangiopancreatography (ERCP). ERCP is a medical procedure that combines an endoscopy with fluoroscopy to diagnose and treat problems of the biliary or pancreatic ducts. **Pancreas cancers** are aggressive types of adenocarcinomas that require complete surgical resection for a chance of cure. If these tumors are *resectable* then a pancreatoduodenectomy (Whipple procedure) is done for cancer of the pancreatic head; otherwise, a distal pancreatectomy is used for tumors of the pancreatic body or tail. Due to its inherent invasiveness, chemotherapy with or without radiation therapy will be recommended for almost all pancreatic cancers even after a successful surgery. If pancreas tumors involve nearby blood vessels, like the superior mesenteric artery or portal vein, they may be borderline resectable or unresectable (not able to safely remove surgically). Chemotherapy or chemoradiation may be used prior to surgery for *borderline resectable* tumors or as definitive treatment for *unresectable* tumors to improve survival. Effective chemotherapy regimens for pancreas cancer may consist of FOLFIRINOX (a chemotherapy regimen of four drugs: leucovorin, fluorouracil (5-FU), irinotecan, and oxaliplatin) or a two-drug regimen of gemcitabine combined with either paclitaxel or capecitabine.

Another major organ of the GI tract, the liver, filters the blood from the digestive tract, detoxifies chemicals, metabolizes drugs, secretes bile, makes proteins important for blood clotting and other functions. Symptoms of **liver cancer** include general GI symptoms in addition to upper abdominal pain, bloating, abdominal swelling (fluid in the abdomen), itching, yellow skin and eyes (jaundice), or white, chalky stools. Along with the standard GI workup, liver tumor workup should include an MRI with contrast and the following laboratory tests: hepatitis panel, bilirubin, transaminases, alkaline phosphatase, PT/INR, and AFP. Primary liver tumors (tumors that start in the liver) may be benign or malignant. Benign (noncancerous) liver tumors are common, do not spread to other areas of the body, usually don't cause serious problems nor need treatment, and include hemangiomas, focal nodular hyperplasias, and hepatocellular adenomas. The most common form of liver cancer in adults is *hepatocellular carcinoma (HCC)*. HCC may be single tumors or many small cancer nodules throughout the liver and is related to cirrhosis (chronic liver damage). Other malignant primary tumors of the liver area include intrahepatic cholangiocarcinoma (bile duct cancer), angiosarcoma, and hemangiosarcoma. *Secondary* liver cancer (metastatic liver cancer) spread from somewhere else in the body, such as the pancreas, colon, stomach, breast, or lung. In the U.S., secondary (metastatic) liver tumors are more common than primary liver cancer, but the reverse is true in Asia and Africa. Treatment of liver cancers includes a wide range of options, such as partial hepatectomy, liver transplant, ablation or embolization, targeted therapy, immunotherapy, chemotherapy (either systemic or by hepatic artery infusion), and/or radiation therapy, including stereotactic body radiation therapy.

The final part of the GI tract consists of the colon, rectum, and anal canal. Cancer of these three distinct organs is often confused by patients who mistakenly consider them to be the same, but there are important differences. Symptoms of **colorectal cancer** include general GI symptoms in addition to change in bowel habits, blood in stool, change in stool consistency, bowel obstruction, narrow stools, diarrhea or constipation, abdominal cramps, passing excessive amounts of gas, or a feeling that your bowel doesn't empty completely. **Anal cancer** symptoms may also include anal or rectal bleeding, anal pain, a mass or growth that can be felt in the anal canal, and anal itching. Along with the standard GI workup, colorectal tumor workup includes colonoscopy with biopsy, CEA (carcinoembryonic antigen) blood test, and possibly an MRI; however, PET/CT is *not* indicated. Anal cancer workup _does_ include PET/CT as well as an inguinal lymph node evaluation with a fine-needle aspiration (FNA) of enlarged nodes, anoscopy, a gynecological exam for women, and an HIV test (since anal cancer is associated with the HPV virus—a sexually transmitted disease). The reason for these differences is based on both anatomy and how they respond to various treatments—to which we will now explore.

Both **colon cancers** and **rectal cancers** are usually the pathological type of cancer called an adenocarcinoma and are treated by surgical resection, so they are often lumped together as colorectal cancers. While there is not much practical difference for the treatment of *early-stage* colon and rectal cancers, treatment recommendations for more advanced stages do differ significantly. For example, colon and rectal cancers require resection or colectomy (removal of part of the colon) and a lymph node dissection for small cancers; however, higher risk tumors require additional treatment. *High-risk* colon cancers (i.e. T3-4 or lymph node positive, LN+) need postoperative chemotherapy, but they rarely receive radiation therapy because the colon moves within the abdominal cavity making it unable to be precisely targeted for radiation treatment. On the other hand, the distal end of the colorectal tract, the rectum, has a higher propensity for local recurrence and is fixed in place by the surrounding support tissues of the pelvis allowing it to be accurately treated with radiation therapy. Therefore, *locally advanced* rectal cancers (i.e. T3-4 or lymph node positive, LN+) usually receive 5-6 weeks of neoadjuvant chemoradiation followed by surgery and additional chemotherapy after surgery. Chemotherapy regimens may include capecitabine, fluorouracil (5FU), or combinations like FOLFOX (leucovorin, 5-FU, and oxaliplatin) or CAPOX (capecitabine and oxaliplatin).

There are even greater disparities for anal cancers because of the difference in pathology. Nearly all anal cancers are the pathological type of cancer called a squamous cell carcinoma and are much more sensitive to chemoradiation than rectal adenocarcinomas. Chemoradiation alone cures anal squamous cell carcinomas more than 80-85% of the time (more than 4 out of 5 patients) even without surgery. Therefore, surgery for anal cancer may be omitted or reserved for salvage of a cancer recurrence. In contrast, rectal adenocarcinomas need aggressive surgery because chemoradiation alone only cures 15-20% of rectal patients (about 1 out of 5) without surgery. Furthermore, a surgery for anal and low-lying rectal cancer, called an abdominoperineal resection (APR), dramatically impacts quality of life because it requires a permanent colostomy bag.

So, in contrast to rectal cancer, most anal cancer patients don't need an APR nor a permanent colostomy. The chemoradiation treatment for anal cancer involves 5-6 weeks of radiation therapy concurrent with a two-drug chemotherapy regimen consisting of either mitomycin and 5FU, mitomycin and capecitabine, or 5FU and cisplatin.

After treatment, follow-up examinations and scans will be done on a routine basis. Initially, you will be seen about every 3 months, but this will extend to every 6 months after a few years and eventually on an annual basis. Overall, side effects of radiation to the GI tract usually include nausea, vomiting, diarrhea, and fatigue. Chemotherapy side effects may include nausea, vomiting, diarrhea, fatigue, hair loss, neuropathy (nerve damage), and a decrease in blood counts which may cause an increased risk of bleeding or infection. Be sure to discuss any side effects, questions, or concerns with your oncologist, family doctor, and family members. For more on chemotherapy and/or radiation side effects from treatment, please refer to Tables 1 & 2 of Chapter 6 in Part I of this book. For additional information regarding other cancer questions, please visit any of the websites mentioned in the Foreword.

CHAPTER FOUR

GYNECOLOGIC (GYN) CANCER

Gynecological (GYN) cancers include tumors of the uterus, cervix, ovaries, or vulva. These types of cancers are often treated by a special surgeon called a gynecologic oncologist who can also prescribe chemotherapy. Symptoms of GYN cancers include constant fatigue, unexplained weight loss, loss of appetite, persistent indigestion or nausea, abnormal vaginal bleeding, vaginal discharge colored with blood, need to urinate more frequently, change in bowel habits, pain or discomfort in the pelvis or abdominal area—including gas, indigestion, pressure, bloating, and cramps. Workup of GYN cancers includes medical history & physical examination, laboratory tests (like CBC, liver and renal function tests, cancer antigen 125 (CA-125) for ovarian cancer), computed tomography (CT) scan of the chest, abdomen, and pelvis with oral and intravenous contrast, possible exam under anesthesia, and biopsy of any suspicious lesions (i.e. cervical biopsy). Further workup may also include PET/CT scan, ultrasound, and MRI of the pelvis (for indeterminate lesions). Treatment recommendations are based on which organ is involved, the pathologic type of cancer, cancer stage, grade, the number of lymph nodes involved, and the general performance status of the patient. Depending on these specifics, chemotherapy and/or radiation therapy may be given before (neoadjuvant), after (adjuvant), or in place of surgery. We will now examine some cancer treatments for the most common GYN cancers.

The uterus, a hollow muscular organ in the female pelvis, functions to allow a developing fetus to implant in the uterine wall for nourishment prior to birth. **Uterine cancer**, or **endometrial cancer**, involves the body of the uterus and is the most common cancer of the female reproductive organs. It is more common in postmenopausal women and is a common cause of postmenopausal bleeding. Most endometrial cancers are a type of adenocarcinoma called endometrioid cancer. It is usually treated by surgically removing the uterus (i.e. hysterectomy), fallopian tubes (i.e. salpingo-oophorectomy), and often some pelvic lymph nodes. Uterine cancer staging depends on the depth of cancer invasion into the uterus and the extent of spread elsewhere. If the cancer only involved the *inner half* of the uterine wall, especially if it is *low grade* (i.e. slow growing), then hysterectomy is usually the only treatment that is necessary. However, if cancer cells invaded *more than halfway* through the uterine wall, or if it is *high-grade*, additional treatment may be needed. For larger or more aggressive tumors, radiation therapy is recommended after hysterectomy to prevent tumor recurrence. Radiation treatments may be given through external beam radiation and/or internal radiation (called brachytherapy). External beam radiation therapy usually requires about 25 treatments over five weeks to the pelvic area. Brachytherapy is a special procedure where focal (very localized) radiation is delivered with radiation sources that are placed directly within the vaginal canal or the uterus to deliver a high dose of radiation next to the tumor area. This technique typically requires 3-5 outpatient procedures given over 2–3 weeks. Each brachytherapy procedure lasts only 10-15 minutes, but the planning process can require a couple of hours. The actual specifics of this form of radiation treatment depend on whether the patient had a hysterectomy or not. If a patient had a hysterectomy, a plastic applicator called a vaginal cylinder (shaped like a large tampon) is inserted into the vagina by the radiation oncologist. The cylinder is temporarily positioned against the blind end of the upper part of the vaginal canal (i.e. vaginal cuff) for the duration of the brachytherapy treatment and then immediately removed so the patient can return home. An extra boost of radiation is directed toward the vaginal cuff because this area poses the highest risk of hiding residual cancer cells. Brachytherapy following hysterectomy for high-risk uterine cancer further decreases the chance of local cancer recurrence.

The cervix, a cylinder-shaped neck of fibromuscular tissue, connects the vagina and the body of the uterus. **Cervical cancer** is more common in women of child-bearing age and most cervical cancers are squamous cell carcinomas that are strongly associated with the sexual transmission of certain strains of HPV (human papilloma virus). Recent data has shown success in preventing the development of cervical (and other) cancers with the widespread use of HPV vaccines in both boys and girls during adolescence. Small or *early-stage* cervical cancer may be successfully treated surgically with a cone biopsy or hysterectomy with or without sparing the ovaries (Note: sparing at least one ovary prevents early menopause in younger women). More *advanced* cervical cancers (stage IB2, II or greater) that are too large to resect or invade surrounding tissues receive more benefit from concurrent chemoradiation rather than hysterectomy. Chemotherapy is cisplatin-based and delivered alongside external beam radiation therapy over about 5 weeks (about 25 radiation treatments). Following chemoradiation, brachytherapy is used to give more radiation dose, called a radiation "boost", to the area with the most tumor cells. The brachytherapy applicator to treat the cervix and uterus consists of a metal or plastic device, called a tandem and ovoids. This applicator is more involved than the vaginal cylinder used after a hysterectomy for endometrial cancer. Prior to cervical brachytherapy, the physician dilates the cervix and sometimes places a small rubber or plastic device, called a cervical sleeve, inside the uterus to keep it open. Part of the applicator, called the tandem, is temporarily inserted through the cervical sleeve and into the cervix by the physician. Two oblong plastic applicators, called ovoids, are placed beside the cervix in the upper-lateral part of the vaginal canal. Gauze packing or small balloons attached to the applicator are used to push the rectum and bladder away from the radiation source to decrease side effects. Once in place, scans are taken to verify proper placement and the radiation sources are loaded into the applicator. Traditionally, low-dose-rate (LDR) sources required several days to deliver the radiation dose to the cervix; but today, high-dose rate (HDR) sources allow each treatment to be completed in about fifteen minutes. To complete a course of brachytherapy to cancer of the cervix or intact uterus usually requires three to five of these HDR brachytherapy treatments. Ideally, the entire treatment should be completed within a total of 8 weeks from the start of radiation treatment. Similarly, more rare cancers of the vaginal canal are treated with chemoradiation and brachytherapy similar to cervical cancers.

The ovaries, the female reproductive glands on each side of the uterus that produce eggs (ova) for reproduction, are also the main source of the female hormones—estrogen and progesterone. While any of the three kinds of ovarian cells can develop into different types of tumor (epithelial, germ cell, or stromal tumors) with different malignant potential (benign, borderline, or malignant), about 85% to 90% of malignant **ovarian cancers** are epithelial ovarian carcinomas. Ovarian cancers are usually surgically removed in a procedure known as an oophorectomy, which is often performed alongside a hysterectomy. This surgery may remove one (unilateral) or both (bilateral) ovaries depending on the stage of tumor, patient's age, and menstrual status. It is important to note that a bilateral oophorectomy will induce surgical menopause that may cause severe symptoms of hormone withdrawal in young women. Some women opt to spare an ovary to maintain their active hormonal status and prevent effects from early menopause, such as osteoporosis and hot flashes. Following surgery, many cases of ovarian cancer will need chemotherapy treatment depending on the grade, stage, and type of cancer. Chemotherapy for ovarian cancer involves getting three to six rounds (i.e. cycles) of a two-drug combination, usually a platinum compound (cisplatin or carboplatin) and a taxane (paclitaxel or docetaxel) given intravenously every 3 to 4 weeks. Some patients also receive targeted therapies with drugs like bevacizumab. Radiation therapy is also sometimes used to treat resistant tumor masses or for palliation.

The vulva, or outer part of the female genitalia, may also develop cancers that are HPV-related. Like cancers of the cervix and anal areas, **vulvar cancer** is typically a squamous cell carcinoma. Vulvar cancer may be both locally aggressive and spread regionally to nearby lymph nodes. If small, these cancers may be completely resected via a wide-local resection or a partial hemi-vulvectomy (surgical removal of part of the vulva). Larger cancers may require a more extensive surgery, called a total vulvectomy (surgical removal of the entire vulva) with sampling or removal of inguinal lymph nodes. These advanced tumors also usually require postoperative radiation directed toward the pelvis and lymph nodes for maximal chance of cure. If the vulvar cancer is too big to remove with surgery, successful treatment may sometimes be achieved with 5-6 weeks of concurrent chemoradiation.

After treatment, follow-up examinations and scans will be done on a routine basis. Initially, you will be seen about every 3 months, but this will extend to every 6 months after a few years and eventually on an annual basis. As with other cancer treatments, side effects from surgery, chemotherapy, and radiation vary depending on the location of the cancer and the specific treatment regimen used. Be sure to discuss any side effects, questions, or concerns with your oncologist, family doctor, and family members. For more on chemotherapy and/or radiation side effects from treatment, please refer to Tables 1 & 2 of Chapter 6 in Part I of this book. For additional information regarding other cancer questions, please visit any of the websites mentioned in the Foreword.

CHAPTER FIVE

HEAD & NECK CANCERS

S ymptoms of **Head & Neck (H&N) cancer** may include persistent stuffiness of the nose, a mouth ulcer or sore, a lump that doesn't heal, persistent or enlarging lymph node of the neck, a persistent sore throat, unusual ear pain, trouble swallowing, blood in the sputum, hoarseness, or a change in the voice. Head and neck (H&N) cancers are usually squamous cell carcinomas and include tumors of the nasal cavity, nasopharynx (area behind the nasal cavity), oral cavity (buccal mucosa, oral tongue, floor of mouth), oropharynx (tonsils, base of tongue), larynx (supraglottis, glottis, and subglottis), and hypopharynx (pyriform sinus, posterior pharyngeal wall). The first step in treating H&N cancer is to complete a staging workup which typically includes medical history & physical examination—including a complete mirror or fiberoptic H&N exam from an ENT (Ear, Nose & Throat) surgeon, dental evaluation, computed tomography (CT) scan of the neck and chest, and biopsy of any suspicious lesions. Pathologic review of any biopsy specimens should also include immunohistochemical (IHC) stains for the tumor suppressor protein, p16, that is associated with HPV (human papilloma virus) and has been related to more favorable outcomes. Further workup may also include PET/CT scan and/or MRI of the neck to determine the extent of spread.

To highlight the importance of the oncology team and proper staging, let me share a story of one of my patients from several years ago. He was being treated with 7 weeks of chemotherapy and radiation for a H&N cancer that had spread to a couple of regional (nearby) lymph nodes of the neck. Since multiple lymph nodes were involved his lymph node stage was "N2" and overall stage grouping was Stage IVA cancer. (Note: Stage IV Head & Neck cancer is different from other cancers in that it is classified as Stage IV A, B, or C.) His cancer was still considered a regional disease because it had not spread through the blood and he still had a reasonable chance of cure. In fact, I estimated that he had a local control rate of around 70-80% and an overall cure rate better than 50% with combined chemotherapy and radiation. If it had spread to distant organs through the blood (M1), then this H&N cancer would have been assigned Stage IVC and not be considered curable. (Note: This is an exception to the general rules of staging that we previously discussed in Part I.) During treatment, he became dehydrated and needed to get IV fluids in the Emergency Department. Unfortunately, the ER doctor mistook Stage IVA H&N cancer to mean that his cancer had spread through the blood to distant organs and told the family that he was not curable. A very upset patient and family then called me from our hospital's own Emergency Department demanding to know why I had misled them and put him through such a difficult treatment if there was no chance of cure! I dropped what I was doing, immediately marched down the hall, found my patient lying on a gurney, and explained to everyone (including the doctor) that Stage IVA and IVB H&N IS curable with chemo-radiation. It is Stage IVC H&N cancer that has already spread throughout the blood and is, therefore, not curable. This caveat in H&N cancer is tricky because usually the ER doctor's assumption would've been correct—but not in this case. It is important to obtain good information from a reliable source and verify it if you have any doubts.

Treatment depends on which subsite of H&N cancer is involved, size of the tumor, number of lymph nodes involved, tumor HPV status, and general performance status of the patient. While the nuances of surgery and other treatments vary according to these factors, most *early-stage* cancers (T1-2 and N0-1) are often cured by complete resection of the tumor by an ENT surgeon. These oncologic surgeries may or may not include a regional lymph node dissection that may be quite extensive or modified to decrease the risk of side effects, like lymphedema (swelling) or nerve damage. Furthermore, lymph node dissections may be unilateral (one-sided) or bilateral (two-sided) depending on which areas of the neck are at most risk for tumor spread. Some surgeries, like the organ-sparing partial laryngectomy, may be used in some patients with small vocal cord tumors (i.e. T1-2 glottic cancer) to preserve their speaking voice, but a total laryngectomy (i.e. complete removal of the voice box) may be required for larger cancers of the larynx. One organ-sparing approach for small vocal cord tumors is definitive radiation therapy alone to maintain voice quality and still achieve comparable cure rates of 95% (19 out of 20). This daily radiation treatment delivers a small "postage stamp" field over 5-6 weeks to T1 glottic tumors. Another exception where radiation alone is used rather than surgery is in small cancers of the nasopharynx. For larger nasopharynx cancers, chemotherapy and radiation are used together concurrently (i.e. chemoradiation) for best results.

Likewise, *advanced* cancers (T3-4 or multiple positive lymph nodes) of most H&N sites will be treated with either surgery and adjuvant radiation with or without chemotherapy (after visible tumor is surgically removed) or definitive chemoradiation without surgery. Based on the high-risk factors for recurrence, the indications for postoperative radiation are extranodal extension (i.e. tumor that extends outside lymph nodes), positive margin, T3-4 primary, N2-3 nodal disease, and perineural or vascular or lymphatic invasion. For example, if a tonsil (oropharynx) cancer patient presents with two or more enlarged lymph nodes of the neck that "light up" on a preoperative PET/CT, then we already know that this patient will need radiation treatment even before surgery because they have multiple involved lymph nodes and are staged as N2 (IVA). Both adjuvant and definitive chemoradiation for H&N cancer may involve a cisplatin-based chemotherapy regimen delivered every three weeks for a total of three cycles (day 1, 22, and 43) during radiation or a lower dose of chemotherapy given once per week concurrently with radiation treatments. One notable difference between adjuvant (postoperative) radiation versus definitive chemoradiation is the total number of treatments for cure—30-33 fractions over 6 to 6 ½ weeks for the former and 35 fractions over seven weeks for the latter. As you can see, one may avoid the side effects of surgery by only adding a week or less of radiation treatments without losing any chance of cure.

To explain the roles of surgery and chemoradiation in locally advanced H&N cancer, consider how treatment recommendations have changed in recent decades. For many years, an extensive surgical resection to attempt complete removal of H&N cancers was the only available treatment. With advances in less invasive surgical techniques, like TORS (transoral robotic surgery), surgical outcomes improved while decreasing side effects. Meanwhile, radiation therapy (and more recently chemoradiation) has matured from early organ-sparing treatment to widespread use in most H&N cancers. Large, randomized research trials confirmed that chemoradiation could cure most H&N cancers without the need for large, debilitating surgeries. Therefore, treatment recommendations began to shift in the late-1990's from surgery with adjuvant radiation used after surgery to upfront chemotherapy and radiation. Surgery can be reserved as a salvage treatment for later tumor recurrence if necessary. There is still considerable debate among surgeons and other oncologists about the role of surgery in these larger, yet curable, cancers. For example, some good evidence shows that T4 larynx cancers or very large lymph nodes of the neck may still benefit from surgical removal even after a good response from neoadjuvant (upfront) chemoradiation. Nevertheless, because of the curative success of modern chemoradiation in squamous cell carcinoma of H&N cancers, the role of surgery has become less prominent for these responsive tumors in recent years.

Now that we have discussed the symptoms, workup, staging, and treatments for H&N cancer, I want to spend some time explaining what to expect prior to chemoradiation, whether after surgery or as definitive treatment. Most patients are surprised at how many steps are involved prior to starting these treatment regimens. Initially, the patient needs a referral to a dentist to completely remove any bad teeth to decrease the risk of future complications of the jawbone. If several teeth require removal, an urgent referral is usually made to an oral surgeon for extraction. After dental surgery, the gums must be allowed to heal for a week or so prior to the creation of a customized facemask for radiation treatment. The radiation mask fits tightly so any swelling from a dental procedure must resolve or else the mask will be too loose during treatment and the entire plan must be redone—a time-consuming and labor-intensive process. After the mask is created, a 30-minute procedure called a CT simulation is done, and the CT images are transferred digitally to a specialized treatment planning computer. It typically takes about a week for your team of radiation oncologists, medical dosimetrists, and medical physicists to create, analyze, and verify the accuracy of a radiation treatment plan. Only after an extensive quality assurance process is verified and completed is the patient called back to start radiation treatment.

Meanwhile, several other things must be coordinated for most H&N patients. These include a medical oncology consultation to discuss whether a regimen of chemotherapy is needed and, if so, which one. Risks and benefits, side effects, and many other things are discussed during this initial visit with the chemotherapy doctor. To deliver chemotherapy, a "port" is usually required and is surgically implanted to give access to the bloodstream. Another surgical device that may be needed is a feeding tube, commonly called a PEG (Percutaneous Endoscopic Gastrostomy) tube. This little rubber tube has a balloon or flange on one end that is placed into the stomach. The other end of the PEG tube is pulled through the abdominal wall (while the patient is under anesthesia) and sticks out of the body. The external end of the tube has a little plastic cap that can be flipped open (like the air nozzle on a pool raft). This allows liquid and food to be squirted directly into the stomach with a syringe. [NOTE: Your body doesn't care how the nutrition gets to the gut, just that it gets there]. Unfortunately, the joy of tasting food is bypassed with a feeding tube, but that won't matter because after a few weeks of radiation treatment, you won't be able to taste anything for several weeks anyway.

Feeding tubes may help H&N patients complete radiation treatment without becoming malnourished and dehydrated. Feeding tubes allow food and water to be given to patients with a sore throat or those unable to swallow due to the side effects of H&N radiation therapy. Dehydration places extra strain on the heart and kidneys and, if severe, can eventually become life threatening. For many years, PEG tubes were inserted before radiation due to fear of performing a surgery during treatment with a swollen airway from radiation and an excess risk of bleeding during chemotherapy. Unfortunately, some recent evidence shows a substantially increased risk of permanent PEG tube dependence by placing tubes earlier rather than later in treatment, particularly if patients aren't diligent in forcing themselves to swallow at least a little bit every day. A recent trend is to hold off on placement of feeding tubes until absolutely necessary, but this should be discussed with your doctor on a case-by-case basis. Radiation usually causes a sore throat by about week three, especially if chemotherapy is also given. Many patients require short and/or long-term narcotic pain medicine to help with swallowing. Even with a feeding tube, patients can work the swallowing muscles by taking small sips of liquid every day. Adding 2-3 protein shakes to supplement meals can help prevent malnourishment. If the patient is not able to eat any meals, then 5-6 cans of protein drinks are necessary each day to maintain an appropriate weight. In place of expensive protein drinks, you may simply add some water to last night's leftovers (especially protein—meat, eggs, cheese, peanut butter, etc.), mix it up in a blender, and inject it in the feeding tube. If a full stomach causes nausea or indigestion, decrease the volume by half and take six small meals throughout the day rather than three bigger meals. The key to successful nutrition during treatment is smaller amounts of food taken more often.

After H&N radiation, the side effects resolve at different rates. Skin redness, sore throat, and fatigue mostly resolve about a month after the last radiation treatment. The loss of taste recovers after a couple of months. Taste sensations return at different rates with bitter and sour recovering earlier than sweet tastes. Radiation causes a dry mouth (called xerostomia) and thick saliva that slowly improves over 3-12 months but expect some dryness to be permanent. Modern radiation, like Intensity-Modulated Radiation Therapy (IMRT), may spare a good portion of the salivary glands, particularly the parotid glands, from permanent dryness but they are still "stunned" and it takes a while for them to recover. Follow-up appointments will focus on resolution of symptoms. Future laryngoscopies by the ENT physician and occasional CT scans will monitor for recurrence. These exams are more frequent for the first couple of years and then less often as time passes. For more on chemotherapy and/or radiation side effects from treatment, please refer to Tables 1 & 2 of Chapter 6 in Part I of this book. For additional information regarding other cancer questions, please visit any of the websites mentioned in the Foreword.

CHAPTER SIX

LUNG AND THORACIC CANCER

Thoracic cancers are tumors of the chest that include lung cancer, malignant mesothelioma, thymus cancer, and lymphomas. The primary focus of this chapter will be on cancers that originate directly from the lung tissue. Lung cancer is an aggressive tumor that starts in the lung and often spreads to nearby lymph nodes in the middle of the chest or to distant organs through the bloodstream, such as the brain, liver, bones, and/or other parts of the lung. Lymphomas are addressed in the next chapter.

Symptoms of lung or thoracic cancers may include cough (often with blood), hoarseness, chest pain, shortness of breath, wheezing, fatigue, swollen lymph nodes, weakness, loss of appetite, or weight loss. Occasionally, these symptoms will not appear until the cancer is advanced. Before treatment options can be recommended, a workup must be done to determine if cancer cells have spread to other areas of the body. Workup typically involves a medical history and physical examination, CBC and routine blood tests, CT scan of the chest, PET/CT of the body, and MRI of the brain. Tumors of the chest usually require a visual inspection of the airway by a lung doctor (pulmonologist) with the use of a flexible light with a camera, called a bronchoscope. Since some lung tumors spread to the nearby lymph node area of the chest, called the mediastinum, a surgical procedure may be required to complete the staging workup. Some bronchoscopes are equipped with an ultrasound, called an endobronchial ultrasound (EBUS), that allow evaluation of the mediastinal lymph nodes. A more invasive surgical procedure, called a mediastinoscopy, may also be recommended. A mediastinoscopy removes a few of the many lymph nodes located above the heart where the root of the lung, aorta, and pulmonary arteries come together. This collecting area is a common location where infections or tumors spread and an EBUS or mediastinoscopy may help doctors decide whether to recommend a larger surgery to remove a lobe of the lung (lobectomy) or not.

The two major types of lung cancer are **small cell lung cancers (SCLC)** and **non-small cell lung cancers (NSCLC)**. SCLC make up less than 20% of all lung cancers and are very likely to spread through the blood even before the patient knows they have cancer. It is best treated with chemotherapy and radiation to the lung and brain. The treatment and prognosis of SCLC is very different than NSCLC and it is considered a completely different disease. Surgery is not a routine part of treatment for SCLC. It may be counterintuitive, but even though SCLC responds better to chemotherapy and radiation therapy than NSCLC, it has a worse prognosis due to its propensity to spread. The stage of SCLC is less important than in NSCLC because its treatment is based more on its response to chemotherapy.

The remaining 80% of lung cancers are classified together as NSCLC because they are all treated in a similar fashion. The group of NSCLCs is quite diverse, made up of subgroups such as adenocarcinomas, squamous cell carcinomas, and large cell carcinomas. Generally, there are 3 different treatment scenarios for NSCLC: early-stage, locally advanced, and metastatic lung cancer.

The first scenario involves *early-stage* NSCLC (T1-2 and N0-1—overall stage group I or II) that are small and have little or no spread to nearby lymph nodes and are best treated with resection of that part of the lung, called a lobectomy. Recent surgical developments, such as sub-lobar lobectomies have had encouraging results in patients with poor lung function that may not be candidates for removal of an entire lobe of the lung. If the patient is not a candidate for any type of curative lung surgery (due to poor heart or lung function), a powerful, non-invasive treatment has become commonplace over the last decade that uses very high doses of pinpoint radiation to ablate or kill small tumors throughout the body, including lung tumors. This advanced technique, called Stereotactic Body Radiation Therapy (SBRT) kills the tumor at that location (i.e. a local cure at the site of tumor) in over 90% of cases. At this point, patients eligible for surgery should consider having it cut out, but there is now an excellent alternative treatment for those that can't or don't want to have surgery. Ultimately, the cure rate for stage I NSCLC is around 50% because of the risk of undetected microscopic tumor cells that might have spread before treatment. Since lung cancers generally grow faster than slower cancers, like prostate cancer, any recurrences of lung cancer are most likely to appear in the first 2–3 years after treatment. Nevertheless, you won't really know if you're cured until about 5 years or so down the road when no signs of cancer can be seen on CT, PET/CT, and MRI scans.

The second scenario includes *locally-advanced* NSCLC (T3-4 or N2-3—overall stage group III) that are larger and/or have spread to the nearby mediastinal lymph nodes in the center of the chest. If a tumor has spread to the mediastinal lymph nodes, surgical resection may still be possible; however, most patients undergo concurrent chemotherapy and radiation (chemo-radiation) instead of surgery. Chemotherapy typically involves a platinum chemotherapy (cisplatin-based) paired with another drug and sometimes an immunotherapy. Radiation focused on the tumor and lymph nodes typically lasts about 6 weeks and is given over about 30 treatments concurrently with chemotherapy treatment. Recently, a new class of biologic agents called checkpoint inhibitor drugs, like durvalumab, has shown to benefit this group of patients when taken after chemoradiation for up to one year. Typical side effects from chemotherapy include fatigue, hearing loss, some loss of kidney function, temporary confusion ("chemo-brain"), temporary drop in blood counts, as well as tingling and loss of sensation in the fingers and toes (paresthesia and neuropathy). Radiation therapy side effects include fatigue, permanent scarring of the area of lung where the tumor is located (other areas of the lung are unaffected), sore throat/esophagitis (if the tumor is close to the center of the chest or mediastinal lymph nodes are treated), and sometimes temporary redness (erythema) of the skin over the chest and back.

The third scenario of NSCLC patients is with *metastatic* (Stage IV) disease that has spread to other parts of the body. Unfortunately, Stage IV lung cancer is not usually curable but that does NOT mean that it isn't treatable. Recent genetic tests have identified some subgroups of NSCLC with certain genetic changes, such as ALK or EGFR mutations, that have significantly better outcomes than other lung cancers. Often chemotherapy and newer biologic agents, like immunotherapy (nivolumab, ipilimumab, etc.) are used to slow or shrink cancers. Radiation therapy is specifically used to extend survival in lung cancers that have spread to the brain and can be either whole-brain treatments or very focal, short-course treatments. Radiation can also be effective in improving quality of life by preventing rib or bone pain, bleeding, fractures, or other potential tumor-related problems. Remember that palliative treatments often help many people live longer and have better quality lives, even if the tumor is not curable.

After treatment for SCLC or any of the three scenarios of NSCLC described above, follow-up examinations and scans will be done on a routine basis. Initially, you will be seen about every 3 months, but this will extend to every 6 months after a few years and eventually on an annual basis. There are other differences in treating lung cancer that are beyond the scope of this book so be sure to discuss any side effects, questions, or concerns with your oncologist, family doctor, and family members. For more on chemotherapy and/or radiation side effects from treatment, please refer to Tables 1 & 2 of Chapter 6 in Part I of this book. For additional information regarding other cancer questions, please visit any of the websites mentioned in the Foreword.

CHAPTER SEVEN

LYMPHOMAS, LEUKEMIAS, AND MULTIPLE MYELOMA

The body's immune system fights against infections with the help of special "infection-fighting" cells known as white blood cells (i.e. leukocytes). There are several types of white blood cells, including lymphocytes, macrophages, granulocytes, and monocytes that each make up part of a very complicated system to defend the body against germs. Cancer may develop from any of these cells and it is not surprising that cancers of the immune system are complicated and confusing.

Cancers that originate from the cells of lymph nodes are called lymphomas and are divided into two main types: Hodgkin's Lymphoma (HL) and Non-Hodgkin's Lymphoma (NHL). HL is marked by the presence of characteristic "Reed-Sternberg" cells under a microscope, while NHL do not have these distinctive cells. Cancers that grow from blood-forming cells of the bone marrow are most commonly leukemias or multiple myeloma, but there are many other types of blood-borne cancers.

Symptoms of lymphomas, leukemias, or multiple myeloma may include fever without infection, enlarged lymph nodes, alcohol intolerance, pruritis (itching), easy bruising, bleeding, or special predictive symptoms called "B symptoms" that consist of fever, drenching night sweats, and unintentional weight loss. Workup for these cancers begins with a medical history and physical examination that includes assessment of performance status, splenic exam, and a testicular exam for males. Laboratory tests include standard tests like CBC, platelets, comprehensive metabolic panel, liver function tests; and more specific lab tests such as erythrocyte sedimentation rate (ESR), disseminated intravascular coagulation (DIC) panel [d-dimer, fibrinogen, prothrombin time (PT), partial thromboplastin time (PTT)], tumor lysis syndrome panel, urinalysis, Hepatitis B/C, HIV, CMV Ab testing, and a pregnancy test, if indicated. For multiple myeloma, lab tests also include a serum albumin, uric acid, LDH, free light chain (FLC) assay, beta-2 microglobulin, 24-hour urine for total protein, urine protein electrophoresis (UPEP), and urine immunofixation electrophoresis (UIFE). CT scans with IV and oral contrast and/or a PET/CT of the body are often important in the staging workup, and patient's symptoms may sometimes warrant an MRI of the brain.

Depending on the type of cancer, workup may also include a lumbar puncture (i.e. spinal tap), an echocardiogram or cardiac nuclear medicine scan, and a bone marrow core biopsy with aspirate analysis [including immunophenotyping and cytochemistry to test chromosomes (DNA) using advanced cytogenetics with fluorescent in situ hybridization (FISH) and polymerase chain reaction (PCR)]. The classification of cancers of the immune system and the many specialized tests used to differentiate them is very complicated and further explanation is beyond the scope of this book.

Cancer staging of the immune system, particularly lymphomas, is an important part of describing how much cancer is in the body and in determining prognosis and treatment options. The current staging system for lymphomas is known as the Lugano classification and describes limited stage lymphomas as Stage I or II and more advanced lymphomas as Stage III or IV. If organs outside the lymphatic system are involved with cancer, then they are labeled with an "E" for "extranodal" organs (e.g. stage IE or IIE). Stage I lymphoma involves one lymph node or extranodal area; whereas stage II lymphoma involves two or more lymph nodes or extranodal areas on the same side of the diaphragm (i.e. either both "above" *or* both "below" the thin muscle that separates the chest and abdomen). Stage III lymphoma involves lymph node areas on both sides of (above *and* below) the diaphragm and may also include the spleen. Stage IV lymphoma has spread throughout the body into places such as the bone marrow, liver, or lung. Another staging term, "bulky disease", is used for chest lymphomas greater than one-third of the width of the chest or greater than 10 centimeters in size. Note: Bulky tumors are often treated with radiation therapy after systemic (chemo or biological) therapy.

Typically, **Hodgkin's lymphoma (HL)** affects children and younger adults, involves B lymphocytes, and consists of a variety of subtypes that have different patterns of spread and treatment options. HL usually responds well to chemotherapy and may be grouped as favorable or unfavorable based on its size, number of involved areas, specific lab tests (i.e. ESR < 50 mm/hr is favorable), and its response to chemotherapy. The response of HL to chemotherapy, like other lymphomas, is reevaluated with a restaging PET/CT scan. A lymphoma's response is measured by how much residual uptake is seen on the PET/CT scan and given a Deauville score of one (1) to five (5). Deauville scores of 1–3 indicate a good response, while scores of 4-5 indicate an incomplete response to chemotherapy. While there are several chemotherapy regimens, the most common combination for HL includes the drugs—doxorubicin, bleomycin, vinblastine, and dacarbazine, often called "ABVD".

New biologic drugs and other chemotherapy regimens exist, and treatment recommendations will likely continue to change as ongoing research advances in the future. An example of an exciting new class of drug that oncologists currently use for some high-risk or recurrent HLs is an anti-CD30 antibody that acts like a homing signal for chemotherapy to target the cancer cells. Radiation therapy may also be given after a chemotherapy regimen for early-stage, bulky, or unfavorable disease. The relative five-year survival rate for patients diagnosed with HL is now over 85%, but varies by type, stage, and treatment.

Non-Hodgkin's Lymphomas (NHLs) consist of many different types of cancer, but the two main groups are *B-cell lymphomas* and *T-cell lymphomas*. B-cell lymphomas originate from B lymphocytes that produce antibodies to protect against bacteria or viruses and make up about 85% of lymphomas. T-cell lymphomas arise from T lymphocytes that destroy germs or boost other immune cells and comprise the remaining 15% of lymphomas. The World Health Organization (WHO) designed a classification system for lymphomas that is based on a host of biologic and genetic factors to help describe NHLs as indolent (i.e. slow growing), like follicular lymphoma; or aggressive (i.e. fast growing), like diffuse large B-cell lymphoma (DLBCL).

Diffuse large B-cell lymphoma (DLBCL) is the most common type of NHL in the United States, generally affects older patients, and responds well to treatment. Many patients are permanently cured with chemotherapy regimens like "RCHOP", a combination of an immunotherapy drug, rituximab, and four chemotherapy drugs—cyclophosphamide, doxorubicin, vincristine, and prednisone. The RCHOP regimen is given over 3-6 cycles depending on a patient's stage and risk factors. Radiation therapy may be added for early-stage DLBCL, tumors with less than a complete response to immunochemotherapy (Deauville 4-5), or for palliation.

Paradoxically, patients with indolent lymphomas also respond well to most treatments and may live a long time but are usually *not* as likely to be cured with standard treatments because the tumor often involves the bone marrow. Moreover, sometimes tumors, like follicular lymphomas, can transform into fast-growing tumors, like diffuse large B-cell lymphomas. There are many other distinct NHLs including *mantle cell lymphoma, marginal zone B-cell or MALT lymphomas, primary central nervous system (CNS) lymphoma, primary cutaneous lymphomas (i.e. mycosis fungoides)*, etc.

Leukemias are a class of cancers that originate from the blood and bone marrow, but the line between lymphomas and leukemias is sometimes blurred. Leukemias grow inside the bone marrow cavity and crowd out healthy blood cells, thus weakening the immune system. They may be classified as acute or chronic and include examples like *acute lymphoblastic leukemia (ALL), acute myeloid leukemia (AML), chronic lymphocytic leukemia (CLL), chronic myeloid leukemia (CML)*, and others with varied origins, characteristics, prognosis, and treatments that are beyond the scope of this chapter.

Treatment for lymphomas and leukemias include a wide range of chemotherapy and novel biological therapies. Some systemic therapies include longstanding treatments such as alkylating agents, corticosteroids, platinum drugs, purine analogs, anti-metabolites, anthracyclines, and others. New biological therapies include antibodies that target cancer proteins (i.e. rituximab), immune checkpoint inhibitors (i.e. nivolumab and pembrolizumab), proteasome inhibitors (i.e. bortezomib), histone deacetylase inhibitors (i.e. romidepsin), and tyrosine kinase inhibitors, or TKIs (i.e. dasatinib and imatinib). For tumors that spread to the central nervous system (i.e. brain and spinal cord), treatment with intrathecal chemotherapy (i.e. methotrexate and cytarabine) may be delivered directly into the cerebrospinal fluid (CSF).

Multiple myeloma is a cancer that starts within a type of white blood cell, called plasma cells, that make antibodies (i.e. immunoglobulins) to fight infections. If the tumor only involves one location, it is called a **solitary plasmacytoma** and is sometimes cured with either radiation therapy or surgery. More often, these plasmacytomas spread to multiple locations or involve a person's bone marrow and are called multiple myeloma. Tumors of the plasma cells include a spectrum of diseases (i.e. systemic light chain amyloidosis, Waldenstrom's Macroglobulinemia, etc.) that may be clinically indolent (i.e. smoldering or asymptomatic) or aggressive. Smoldering myeloma may not initially need primary treatment since the disease may not progress for many months or years. More aggressive (i.e. active or symptomatic) myeloma may produce abnormal proteins that can be detected in the blood or urine and sometimes cause complications in the bones, kidneys, or other organs of the body. While generally not curable, active multiple myeloma may be treated with bisphosphonates or denosumab to slow tumor growth, relieve symptoms, and assess tumor response. Primary treatment for myelomas that respond may include induction (i.e. upfront) chemotherapy followed immediately by high-dose therapy or a stem cell transplant. Induction chemotherapy often involves a three-drug regimen of bortezomib, lenalidomide, and dexamethasone, but there are many different drug regimens depending on whether the patient is a candidate for stem cell transplant as well as other factors. Following primary treatment, maintenance therapy with lenalidomide or other similar drugs may be given to slow or prevent recurrence.

Your oncologist will schedule follow-up examinations, lab tests, and scans on a routine basis after treatment for cancers like lymphomas, leukemias, and multiple myeloma. Initially, you will be seen more often—probably every three months or so, but appointments may be spread out if you are doing well. Further details of these complicated cancers are beyond the scope of this booklet so be sure to discuss any side effects, questions, or concerns with your medical oncologist. For more on chemotherapy and/or radiation side effects from treatment, please refer to Tables 1 & 2 of Chapter 6 in Part I of this book. For additional information regarding other cancer questions, please visit any of the websites mentioned in the Foreword.

CHAPTER EIGHT

PROSTATE AND GENITOURINARY (GU) CANCER

Genitourinary (GU) cancers involve tumors of the urinary tract (i.e. kidneys, ureters, bladder, and urethra) or male reproductive organs (i.e. prostate, penis, and testicles). While kidney, bladder, and testicular cancers are more common than some cancers, prostate cancer is far more prevalent than all the other GU cancers combined. In fact, prostate cancer is the most common cancer in men (affecting 1 out of 6 American men) and will be the sole focus of this chapter.

Prostate cancer may present with symptoms like difficulty with urination, frequent urge to urinate, blood in semen or painful ejaculation, but most times there are no symptoms at all. Doctors may order a screening test, called the prostate-specific antigen (PSA) test, to measure the level of PSA in the blood in search of prostate cancer cells. PSA is a protein produced by a man's prostate gland that may be elevated from prostate cancer cells or also from noncancerous conditions such as inflammation of the prostate (prostatitis) and enlargement of the prostate (benign prostatic hyperplasia). A digital rectal exam (DRE), when a doctor feels the prostate for lumps or unusual growths, is also a part of routine screenings and are also important. If abnormalities are suspected on PSA or DRE, an ultrasound with biopsy is usually performed. As typical of any biopsy, ultrasound-guided trans-rectal biopsies of the prostate gland remove small amounts of tissue to microscopically examine for the presence of cancer cells. By far, most prostate cancers are adenocarcinomas. They are staged like any other cancer, but are also classified into risk groups—low, intermediate, and high-risk, by its chance of spreading elsewhere in the body. Stage looks at where the cancer is in your body, but grade describes how the cancer cells look and behave under a microscope (i.e. aggressiveness). To interpret the results from a prostate biopsy, we must explore the Gleason Score and ISUP Grade Group.

These risk groupings have been validated by thousands of patients over several decades and help determine prognosis and treatment options. The Gleason score, named for the pathologist who developed it, groups prostate cancer cells into 5 distinct patterns as they change from normal cells to tumor cells. They are graded from least aggressive to most aggressive on a scale from 1 (normal prostate cells) to 5 ("high-grade" cancer cells that mutated to barely resemble normal cells). The pathologist assigns a Gleason score to the most predominant pattern and the second most predominant pattern in your biopsy and both scores are added together to determine your total Gleason score. While total Gleason scores may technically range from 2–10; most pathologists only assigned scores from 6 to 10, with 6 being the least aggressive grade cancer. Note: any amount of Gleason grade 5 prostate cancer cells puts you at a higher risk of recurrence. Recently, a group of urological pathologists developed a revised prostate cancer grading system, called the ISUP Grade Groups to better classify prostate cancer cells. The ISUP Grade Group system is simpler, with just five grades, 1 through 5, as shown in the table below:

Table 3. Prostate Cancer Risk Groups and ISUP Grade Groups

- Risk Group: Low | ISUP Grade Group 1 | Gleason Score ≤ 6
- Risk Group: Intermediate Favorable | ISUP Grade Group 2 | Gleason Score 7 (3 + 4)
- Risk Group: Intermediate Unfavorable | ISUP Grade Group 3 | Gleason Score 7 (4 + 3)
- Risk Group: High | ISUP Grade Group 4 | Gleason Score 8
- Risk Group: High | ISUP Grade Group 5 | Gleason Score 9-10

After a biopsy confirms the presence of prostate cancer, other medical scans may be ordered. These imaging tests may include a CT scan of the abdomen and pelvis with IV and oral contrast and/or MRI of the prostate. These scans may help determine the size and stage of the cancer. If cancer spread is suspected, whole-body bone scans or PET/CT scans may be ordered to rule out or confirm metastasis. Newer tests that incorporate advanced protein or genomic (DNA) testing are in use at various stages and currently being studied.

While it is true that most men *with* prostate cancer do not die *from* it, prostate cancer still kills many men due to the vast number of cases. The claim that urologists and oncologists have "over-treated" prostate cancer in recent decades highlights the need to determine which prostate cancers really need treatment. When my dad was diagnosed with prostate cancer a few years ago, I remember helping him sort through many different treatment options. He eventually chose a combination of external beam radiation therapy with brachytherapy boost and was pleased with his outcome. Not only was he cured, but his side effects were very minimal. It can be overwhelming, but my advice is that you take your time, learn about your prostate cancer risk group and discover your options.

Low-risk prostate cancer patients are those with small or no prostate nodules, PSA less than 10 ng/mL, and ISUP Group Grade 1 (i.e. Gleason score of 6). The odds of being alive and without evidence of prostate cancer (i.e. normal PSA) with low-risk disease after treatment is about 95% or better at 10 years. Treatment options for low-risk patients include active surveillance (close monitoring of PSA without delivering treatment), traditional external beam radiation therapy (40-45 treatments over 8-9 weeks), moderately hypofractionated (larger doses of radiation in less number of treatments) external radiation therapy (20-30 treatments over 4-6 weeks), extreme hypofractionation with Stereotactic Body Radiation Therapy (SBRT: 5 treatments over 2 weeks), prostate brachytherapy (radiation implant inside the prostate), or radical prostatectomy.

There is much written about these treatment options, but the main point is that they are all acceptable and have overall survival rates that are generally about the same. Results like PSA control rates, disease-free survival, rate of distant metastasis, however, may differ slightly. Despite similar tumor outcomes, these treatments have distinct side effect profiles. For example, active surveillance has no side effects, but may have a higher risk of PSA progression in the future even if it doesn't affect overall survival. External beam radiation therapy has higher quality of life during and after treatment than other treatment options and much less toxicity than in years past. Traditional side effects typically involved gastrointestinal (GI) symptoms, such as diarrhea, nausea, or radiation proctitis, and/or genitourinary (GU) symptoms, such as bladder irritation, urinary frequency, or dysuria (temporary burning with urination). Prostate seed-implant (brachytherapy) delivers a much higher dose than external beam radiation and has been shown in some studies to have extremely high cure rates but may have slightly more bladder irritation and temporary dysuria (burning with urination). Finally, radical prostatectomy removes the entire prostate and part of the urethra while attempting to spare the nerves around the prostate to minimize the risk of erectile dysfunction (ED). While it can occur following any of the definitive treatments, the rate of ED is highest in prostatectomy patients and is highly surgeon dependent. Another side effect that is almost always unique to surgical prostatectomy is urinary incontinence that is worsened with coughing or increased abdominal pressure.

Intermediate-risk prostate cancer patients have either slightly larger tumors, PSA between 10-20 ng/mL, or ISUP Group Grade 2–3 (i.e. Gleason 7 adenocarcinoma). Much has been written recently about Gleason 7 prostate cancer and the variable outcomes within this group. To tease more information out of this pathologic ranking, the ISUP Grade Group classifies Gleason 7 disease as either Group 2 (Gleason 3+4) or Group 3 (Gleason 4+3 disease). *Intermediate favorable* (Group 2) tumors are considered less aggressive than *intermediate unfavorable* (Group 3) prostate cancers. Some doctors will treat Group 2 patients like low-risk cancer and Group 3 patients more like high-risk prostate cancer.

So how does this risk of spread impact cancer treatment? Treatment options for Group 2–3 (intermediate risk) patients include the same treatments listed for low-risk patients, but active surveillance may be recommended less often than definitive treatment. Overall, the chance of being alive and without evidence of prostate cancer after definitive treatment for intermediate-risk prostate cancer is around 85-95%. It is a matter of debate how oncologists and urologists interpret the research data. Many consider Group 2 (intermediate favorable risk) patients to have truly local disease and do not typically treat the pelvic lymph nodes. Conversely, Group 3 (intermediate unfavorable risk) and Group 4-5 (high-risk patients) are more likely to receive radiation or resection (surgical removal) of the pelvic lymph nodes.

For example, consider how a risk group might affect radiation treatment—that is "big-field" versus "little-field" radiation. Big fields treat pelvic lymph nodes to a medium dose and the prostate to a high dose of radiation, while little fields only treat the prostate area to the high dose of radiation. Obviously, treating a larger area with radiation therapy will increase the amount of normal tissue within the treatment field and therefore increase the risk of side effects. Does the benefit outweigh the risk? While the increase in side effects is modest, so might be the benefit. There is conflicting data about whether to treat these pelvic lymph nodes and the consensus opinion among oncologists have shifted back and forth in recent years. Either way, if there is a benefit it is not a large one. I recommend a thorough discussion with your doctor.

A second major impact of risk grouping is whether a patient receives hormonal therapy, or androgen deprivation therapy (ADT), and for how long. It has been known for many decades that the presence of testosterone (the male hormone produced by the testicles) accelerates prostate cancer growth. Lower risk patients don't need hormonal treatment, but higher risk patients benefit when hormone therapy is added to some forms of radiation therapy. The hormone drugs most commonly used today are leuprolide and bicalutamide. Leuprolide is delivered as an injection and is slowly absorbed by the body over several months. Leuprolide belongs to a class of medicine, called gonadotropin releasing hormones (GnRH), that overstimulates the body's own production of hormones and causes a reduction of testosterone in men. Bicalutamide is administered in pill form and is usually taken by mouth daily for several months. Bicalutamide is a type of hormone drug called an antiandrogen, or androgen antagonist, that blocks testosterone receptors and/or testosterone production. Treatment with hormonal therapy generally puts the cancer to sleep (hibernation) for several months up to a couple of years. Hormonal therapy is also sometimes used to shrink the prostate gland prior to treatment, decrease the PSA, decrease cancer spreading, or in metastatic disease. A particularly expedient use of hormonal therapy is to put the cancer on hold and prevent further spread, thus giving a patient more time to explore his treatment options. For intermediate risk prostate cancer, most oncologists recommend four to six months of hormonal (androgen deprivation) therapy.

High-risk prostate cancer patients have larger primary tumors (invading surrounding tissue), PSA greater than 20, or ISUP Group Grade 4-5 (i.e. Gleason score 8-10). Treatment options include those already listed; however, the risk of cancer spread to pelvic lymph nodes is more likely. Many radiation oncologists, but not all, treat the pelvic lymph nodes ("big field" radiation treatment) while treating the prostate and seminal vesicles. Recent studies have shown excellent results and increased cure rates with prostate brachytherapy ("seed implant") used to boost radiation dose to the prostate after external beam radiation to the pelvic area. Prior to external radiation, many oncologists also recommend 2–3 months of upfront (neoadjuvant) hormonal therapy to shrink the prostate and enhance the sensitivity of the cancer cells to radiation. As we discussed above, hormonal (androgen deprivation) therapy is typically given via a daily oral dose of bicalutamide for four to six months and a series of leuprolide injections (2–3 months prior to, during, and following a course of radiation therapy) for a total of one to three years. Of note, recent data suggests that patients with ISUP Group Grade 5 (i.e. Gleason scores of 9-10) may benefit from lifelong hormonal therapy. The use and duration of hormone therapy warrants an in-depth discussion with your oncologist and urologist. There are many possible side effects of hormonal treatments, including hot flashes, erectile dysfunction, loss of interest in sex, bone fractures, loss of bone density, loss of muscle mass, changes in blood lipids, and possible impact on the risk of heart disease. The long-term chance of being alive without evidence of prostate cancer for these patients averages around 65-70%, but there are many studies that show a wider range of results. A handful of studies using external beam radiation to the pelvis and high-dose brachytherapy boost to the prostate have even reported long-term cures above 85% for high-risk prostate cancer patients, although confirmatory studies are currently underway.

Many treatment options also exist today for *metastatic* and/or *recurrent* prostate cancer. For disease that has metastasized to other parts of the body, hormone therapy (androgen deprivation therapy) is often used with good results. As we discussed above, hormonal therapy blocks or prevents testosterone from stimulating prostate cancer cells and can be used to slow the spread of cancer or relieve a patient's symptoms. In addition to antiandrogens like bicalutamide, enzalutamide, and apalutamide, there are novel drugs like abiraterone, and chemotherapy such as docetaxel, that are available to treat metastatic or hormone refractory prostate cancer. For cancer that recurs only in the pelvis following a prostatectomy, salvage radiation therapy may still provide a reasonable chance of cure. For locally recurrent prostate cancer following radiation therapy, treatments such as salvage radical prostatectomy, cryotherapy, high-intensity focused ultrasound (HIFU), prostate brachytherapy, or hormonal therapy may be considered.

After treatment for any of the scenarios described above, follow-up examinations, PSA tests, and possibly scans will be done on a routine basis. Initially, you will be seen about every 3 months, but this will extend to every 6 months after a few years and eventually to an annual basis. The variety of treatment options can make deciding how to deal with prostate cancer particularly frustrating for many patients. Talk to friends and family that have undergone the different procedures and ask about side effects. You have time to make the best decision for you. If you need more than a few weeks to come to your decision, ask your urologist to prescribe a short-term hormonal therapy to put the cancer to sleep for a few months while you gather more information. Take time to sort through the options and seek advice from a radiation oncologist and your urologist. Do your homework and go with your gut. For more on radiation side effects from treatment, please refer to Table 2 of Chapter 6 in Part I of this book. For additional information regarding cancers of the prostate or GU tract, or for answers to other cancer questions, please visit any of the websites mentioned in the Foreword.

CHAPTER NINE

SKIN CANCER

Skin cancer is the most common cancer in human beings. Fortunately, most skin cancers can be treated quickly and effectively with local surgery. However, there are some skin cancers, like melanoma, that can be deadly. The three most common types of skin cancer (from least to most aggressive) are basal cell carcinomas, squamous cell carcinomas, and melanomas. You and your doctor should routinely examine your skin to look for skin cancers. Signs of skin cancer may begin as an unusual skin growth or sore that doesn't go away. **Basal and squamous cell (non-melanoma) skin cancers** may initially appear as a nodule, rash, or irregular patch on the surface of the skin that may be raised, and itch or bleed easily. *Basal cell carcinomas* may appear as a pale patch of skin or a smooth, pink, red, pearly, or waxy translucent bump, sometimes with blood vessels or an indentation. Other times, it may be a brownish scar or flesh-colored lesion that may sometimes bleed, ooze, or become crusty. *Squamous cell carcinomas* are typically rough, firm lumps, or a reddish, scaly patch that continues to grow slowly. **Melanoma skin cancers** may appear as a mole that changes in color, size, or feel, or that bleeds; a large brownish spot with darker speckles; a small lesion with an irregular border and portions that appear red, pink, white, blue, or blue-black; or a painful lesion that itches or burns. For melanoma, remember the *ABCDE* rule—an acronym to identify an atypical mole or melanoma based on: *A*symmetry, irregular *B*order, multiple or unusual *C*olor, large *D*iameter, and evidence that the mole is *E*volving.

Workup should include a medical history and physical exam, including a complete skin exam. Any suspicious areas should undergo a biopsy to confirm or exclude a diagnosis of cancer. For advanced cases of melanoma, additional workup will be recommended and may include a sentinel lymph node biopsy, CT scans of the chest, abdomen, and pelvis with IV and oral contrast, and possibly a PET/CT scan and/or an MRI of the brain with IV contrast.

Treatment options for non-melanoma skin cancers vary depending on the type, size, and location of the lesion. Noncancerous lesions, like actinic keratoses (i.e. solar keratoses from chronic sun damage) may be treated simply by freezing with liquid nitrogen (cryosurgery). Small skin cancers that are limited to the skin surface may not require treatment beyond an initial skin biopsy that removes the entire growth (excisional surgery with a negative margin). They may also be cured by using a circular blade (curet) and an electric needle to scrape away and destroy any remaining cancer cells (curettage and electrodesiccation) or by using a combination of laser light and light-sensitizing drugs (photodynamic therapy—PDT). A wide excision—removing extra normal skin around the tumor—may be recommended in some cases.

Mohs surgery is a procedure for basal or squamous cell skin cancers that are large, recurring or in difficult-to-treat areas, like around the eyes, ears, nose or mouth. During a Mohs surgery, the surgeon removes the cancer layer by layer in order to conserve as much skin as possible, examining each layer under the microscope, until no cancer cells remain. The local cure rate for Mohs surgery is reported to be greater than 95% (19 out of

20). Another tissue-preserving option includes radiation therapy for difficult-to-resect cancers. Radiation therapy is often used for larger tumors or ones that cannot be completely resected. Results are dependent on size, location, and radiation dose, but are in the range of 90-95% (better than 9 out of 10) even without surgery. Chemotherapy creams or lotions may sometimes be applied directly to shallow skin lesions and systemic chemotherapy or new biological therapies may be used for some widespread, aggressive cancers.

Basal cell carcinomas are relatively slow growing and only very rarely spread elsewhere. Yet, they can destroy local tissues over time and become a problem, particularly if on the head or face. Surgery with wide margins or radiation is often used to achieve local cure rates of at least 95% without too much difficulty. *Squamous cell carcinomas* are a little more aggressive and have up to a 10% risk of spreading to regional lymph nodes. Surgery or radiation are also effective for this type of skin cancer and cure rates are generally higher than 90%. If surgery is done, several weeks of postoperative (adjuvant) radiation therapy is still indicated if surgical margins were positive or the tumor was not completely removed via surgery.

High-risk factors that increase the chance of tumor recurrence include tumors larger than one to two centimeters, tumor depth greater than six millimeters or invasion into surrounding tissues, poorly differentiated or high-grade tumors, high-risk location (i.e. face, genitals, hands, or feet), poorly-defined or irregular borders, invasion of peripheral nerves or lymphatic or vascular tissues, immunosuppressed patients, and a few other factors. If these factors are present in either basal or squamous cell carcinomas, radiation therapy may be recommended to decrease the chance of recurrence even if the tumor margins following surgery were negative. Radiation therapy for skin cancer requires between 5-30 radiation treatments over one to six weeks depending on which radiation treatment regimen is most appropriate for the situation. Radiation side effects may include a temporary sunburn and probably permanent hair loss from any hair follicles within the treatment area. Nevertheless, skin is very resilient and heals within a three to four weeks after treatment.

The most aggressive form of skin cancer is *malignant melanoma*. This type of skin cancer is best treated with a wide excision surgery because it is somewhat resistant to radiation therapy and less sensitive to most forms of chemotherapy. Not all melanomas will spread, but it is unpredictable and certain forms are deadly. The thickness, or depth of invasion, is one of the critical factors that determine the risk of spread and treatment recommendations. For thicker tumors (greater than 1 millimeter) or for melanoma that has spread to regional lymph nodes or elsewhere, further treatment may consist of lymph node dissection, systemic therapies, and sometimes radiation therapy.

Systemic therapy incorporates many new medicines that have shown promise in the past decade. These novel drug therapies include nivolumab, pembrolizumab, dabrafenib/trametinib (for BRAF V600-active mutation), intralesional injection of a modified herpesvirus to attack cancer called talimogene laherparepvec (T-VEC), BCG, interferon, and interleukin-2. A malignant melanoma that is not removed early preferentially spreads to the skin, lung, brain, liver, bone, and intestine—but can grow anywhere in the body. For a malignant melanoma that has spread to the brain, radiation therapy with or without surgery may be effective.

After treatment, follow-up examinations and scans will be done on a routine basis. Initially, you will be seen about every 3 months, but this will extend to every 6 months after a few years and eventually to an annual basis. As with any cancer, skin cancers can vary in aggressiveness, treatment options, and prognosis. While many people are cured from these common cancers, certain types are more serious and require aggressive treatment. Find a physician that you trust and don't be afraid to ask questions if something doesn't make sense to you. For more on chemotherapy and/or radiation side effects from treatment, please refer to Tables 1 & 2 of Chapter 6 in Part I of this book. For additional information regarding other cancer questions, please visit any of the websites mentioned in the Foreword.

PARTING THOUGHTS

A
s stated in the foreword, the goal of this little book is to provide patients and families with a short and general overview of what cancer is, how it behaves, what tests are used, and what treatments are reasonable. There are volumes of books and countless pages on internet websites that describe thousands of important topics in very specific detail—this was not my objective. Besides not being able to carry a book that big, you couldn't read it all. I think it is easy to find yourself bogged down in details, so I find that some basic principles go a long way in helping us understand what to expect. Only when we understand the good and bad of a treatment option can we really make an informed decision about what is best for us. I hope that by sharing some basic cancer principles in Part I and more specific cancer details in Part II I have provided information that will help you in making treatment decisions.

Finally, I am told that facing a diagnosis of cancer can be one of the scariest and shocking challenges that a person can face. Some are rocked to their core; others *appear* to carry on as if merely inconvenienced. Remember—all of this *is* overwhelming, so give yourself a moment to absorb what is happening. A diagnosis of cancer, the information overload of treatment options, the logistics of juggling appointments, the thought of impending side effects, and the fear of cancer recurrence can cause some to forget that they still have a life worth fighting for. When sorting out what to do, especially early on, it really helps to bring a friend or family member with you to help ask questions and take notes. Some have extended families to sit with them, offer rides, and give support, while others feel alone. No matter what situation you find yourself in, know that others have been where you are *now* and still others will be in the *future*. There are helpers in various places—some of them are the angels I have personally worked with over the years. Remember to keep breathing, put one foot in front of the other, and take each day as it comes. I hope to have helped you in some small way and would love to hear your story if you wish to share. God bless you and good luck!

GLOSSARY

ABCDE rule: An acronym for the general guidelines used to identify an atypical mole or melanoma based on the following features: Asymmetry, irregular Border, multiple or unusual Color, large Diameter, and evidence that the mole is Evolving.

Active surveillance: A treatment plan that involves closely watching a patient's condition but not giving any treatment unless there are changes and test results that show the condition getting worse.

Acute side effects: A health problem that occurs quickly or abruptly after a disease is diagnosed or shortly after treatment has ended.

Adenocarcinoma: A cancer formed from glandular structures in epithelial tissue. They are the most common cancer of the breast, salivary glands, stomach, pancreas, bowel (colon & rectum), and prostate gland.

Adjuvant chemotherapy: Chemotherapy given after all known cancer has been surgically removed or after radiation treatment.

APR (Abdominoperineal resection): A surgery for rectal or anal cancer that completely removes the anal canal and results in a permanent colostomy.

Biological therapy or biotherapy: A type of cancer treatment that uses molecules made from living organisms to enhance or block pathways within the body to fight cancer growth; such as immunotherapy, monoclonal antibodies, epidermal growth factor receptor drugs, etc.

Biopsy: The sampling or removal of body tissue for examination under a microscope to check for cancer cells or other abnormalities.

Bone scan or bone scintigraphy: A medical scan to check for abnormal areas of bone or damage to the bones. A very small amount of radioactive material is injected into a vein, travels through the blood, collects in the bones, and is detected by a scanner. A bone scan may be used to diagnose bone tumors or cancer that has spread to the bone but may also show uptake due to fractures or infections.

Brachytherapy: A form of radiation therapy where a sealed radiation source is placed inside a tumor or next to an area of cancer. Brachytherapy is commonly used as an effective treatment for cancers of the cervix, uterus, prostate, breast, esophagus, and skin cancer and can be used to treat tumors in many other body sites.

Brain metastases: Cancer cells that travel through the bloodstream from the original site of cancer and spread to the brain where they multiply, put pressure on the brain, and may cause headache, nausea, neurologic problems, or seizures.

BRCA (BReast CAncer) gene: A class of genes, called tumor suppressor genes, that normally act to restrain the growth of cells in the breast but when mutated predisposes the individual to developing breast cancer.

Breast conservation surgery: See lumpectomy.

Cancer staging: A way to describe how much cancer is in your body and where it is located in your body. Cancer staging may be either *clinical* (using only the information from medical scans) or *pathologic* (using information from both medical scans and staging surgeries, like lymph node dissections) and helps determine where the original tumor is, how big it is, whether it has spread, and where it has spread.

Cancer statistics: The science of collecting, summarizing, presenting and interpreting data in medical practices, specifically regarding cancer patients and their diagnoses, and using them to estimate cure rates and likelihood of survival at different points in time.

CBC (Complete Blood Count): A blood test used to evaluate your overall health and detect a wide range of disorders, including anemia, infection, and leukemia. It measures the cells that make up your blood: red blood cells, white blood cells, and platelets.

CEA (Carcinoembryonic antigen): A blood test for a protein that is used as a tumor marker, most commonly associated with colon and rectal tumors, but also found in a developing fetus and many other types of normal cells.

Chemo-brain or chemo-fog: A common term used by cancer survivors to describe thinking and memory problems that can occur during and after cancer treatment.

Chemotherapy: A drug treatment that uses powerful chemicals to kill fast-growing cells in your body.

Clinical staging: A method that uses only lab tests and medical imaging to describe how much cancer is in a cancer patient's body by defining where the original tumor is located, how big it is, if it has spread, and to where it has spread. Clinical staging may be slightly different from and is *less* accurate than pathologic staging.

Colonoscopy: A procedure whereby a physician inserts a viewing tube (colonoscope) into the rectum for the purpose of inspecting the colon. During colonoscopy, polyps can be removed, bleeding can be cauterized, and a biopsy can be performed if abnormal areas of the colon are seen.

Complete axillary dissection: The removal of lymph nodes from the area of the armpit, or axilla, whereby 10-20 lymph nodes are typically removed at a moderate risk of causing lymphedema of the arm.

Concurrent chemotherapy: The use of chemotherapy delivered during or alongside radiation treatments.

Core needle biopsy: A diagnostic biopsy procedure to remove a piece of tissue from a lesion or mass. The tissue is then tested under a microscope to find out what it is. A core needle biopsy can remove more tissue than a fine needle biopsy and can provide more information about the cells and tissue removed.

CT (Computed Tomography) scan or CAT scan: A medical scan that uses the absorption of X-rays by different tissue densities in 3-dimensions to reveal anatomic details of internal organs that cannot be seen on conventional X-rays. CT scans provide cross-sectional images of the bones, blood vessels, and soft tissues inside your body.

CT simulation or simulation CT scan: A CT scan performed in order to define the radiation therapy fields for radiation treatment planning.

DAI (Diffuse Axonal Injury): A brain injury in which scattered lesions in white matter tracts as well as gray matter occur over a widespread area. It occurs in about half of all cases of severe head trauma and may be the primary damage that occurs in a concussion.

Diagnostic tests: Examinations to determine which disease or condition explains a person's symptoms and signs.

Disease-Free-Survival (DFS): The length of time after treatment during which no disease is found.

DNA (Deoxyribonucleic acid): A macromolecule that is known as the "blueprints of the cell" and one of two types of molecules that encode genetic information.

Dysuria: Pain or discomfort when urinating.

Endoscopic ultrasound (EUS): A minimally invasive medical procedure in which a special endoscope uses high-frequency sound waves (ultrasound) to visualize the walls, lymph nodes, and adjacent tissues of internal organs in the chest, abdomen, or colon to assess GI or lung diseases.

Endoscopy: A surgical procedure used to examine a person's digestive tract with an endoscope, a flexible tube with a light and camera that can also take biopsy samples.

ENT (Ears, Nose, and Throat) surgeon: A medical specialist, also called an otolaryngologist, concerned with the diagnosis and treatment of disorders of the head and neck, particularly the ears, nose, and throat.

Endoscopic retrograde cholangiopancreatography (ERCP): A medical procedure that combines an endoscopy with fluoroscopy to diagnose and treat problems of the biliary or pancreatic ducts.

Epithelial carcinoma: A cancer that begins in the cells that line an organ.

European Organization for Research and Treatment of Cancer (EORTC): A non-profit cancer research organization whose goal is to coordinate and conduct international translational and clinical research to improve the standard of cancer treatment for patients.

Fine-needle aspiration (FNA): A diagnostic biopsy procedure used to investigate lumps, masses, or bodily fluids via a thin, hollow needle that is inserted into the area of abnormal-appearing tissue for sampling of cells that, after being stained, will be examined under a microscope to look for cancer cells and other diseases.

Fraction: A single radiation treatment that is part of a larger treatment plan whereby the total dose of radiation is spread out over multiple, small, equivalent, daily radiation doses.

Frozen section: A rapid analysis that freezes, slices, and microscopically examines a cancer specimen while surgery is underway to determine if all the cancer was removed. It is generally accurate, but not as trustworthy as a permanent section that requires a more time-consuming preparation of the specimen that requires several days after surgery to obtain the final analysis.

Genetic markers: A DNA sequence at a known physical location on a chromosome that can link an inherited disease with a responsible gene and may help estimate the risk of developing cancer in some patients.

Genetic mutations: A permanent change, or structural alteration, in the DNA sequence that makes up a gene and is one of many steps necessary to transform a normal cell into a cancer cell.

Genetic status or Oncotype DX score: The Oncotype DX test is a genetic test that analyzes the activity of a group of 21 genes from a breast cancer tissue sample that can affect how a cancer is likely to behave and respond to treatment. It assigns a Recurrence Score, a number between 0 and 100, to an early-stage breast cancer.

Gleason score: A grading system used to determine the aggressiveness of prostate cancer by analyzing prostate cancer cells under a microscope and assigning a score that ranges from 6-10 (least to most aggressive).

Grade: A pathologic scale that assigns a value of one (1) for the lowest grade cancers (least aggressive, well-differentiated, slower growing), up to three or four (3-4) for the highest grade cancers (most aggressive, poorly differentiated or undifferentiated; faster growing). Tumor grade is determined by a pathologist during a microscopic assessment to evaluate the rate of cell growth (i.e. number of mitosis) and is different from cancer stage.

Gynecologic oncologist: A physician specifically trained to diagnose and treat cancers of the female reproductive system, including the ovaries, uterus, cervix, vagina, and vulva; through the use of both surgery and chemotherapy.

HPV (human papilloma virus): A virus that is the most common sexually transmitted infection (STI), mostly by the late teen years and early 20s. Some types of HPV cause health problems like genital warts and cancers. HPV is different from HIV and herpes viruses.

Hormonal therapy or endocrine therapy: A medical treatment using synthetic or naturally derived hormones or medicines to block hormone receptors to slow or stop the growth of cancer, other diseases, or symptoms.

Hospice programs: Care organizations designed to give supportive care to people in the final phase of a terminal illness and focus on comfort and quality of care, rather than cure. The goal is to enable patients to be comfortable and free of pain, so that they live each day as fully as possible.

Hysterectomy: A surgery to remove the uterus, either via an open surgery or a laparoscopic surgery, and often also includes the removal of the ovaries, fallopian tubes, and the cervix.

ICU (Intensive care unit): A special department of a hospital or health care facility that provides intensive medical treatment and critical medical care.

Image-Guided Radiation Therapy (IGRT): A modern technique using advanced medical imaging or scans during radiation therapy to improve the precision and accuracy of radiation treatment delivery. IGRT allows the safe delivery of high doses of radiation therapy, even to tumors that move within the body, such as with lung or prostate tumors.

Immunotherapy or biologic therapy: A cancer treatment that boosts the body's natural defenses to fight cancer. It uses substances made by the body or in a laboratory to improve or restore immune system function.

Intensity Modulated Radiation Therapy (IMRT): An advanced form of radiation treatment which uses computer-controlled linear accelerators to deliver precise radiation doses to a malignant tumor or specific areas within the tumor while sparing more normal tissues compared with conventional radiotherapy techniques.

Late side effects: A health problem that occurs months or years after a disease is diagnosed or after treatment has ended. Late effects may result from cancer or cancer treatment and may include physical or mental problems or secondary cancers.

Linear accelerator (Linac): A man-made machine that uses microwave technology to accelerate electrons to collide with a heavy metal target and produce high-energy X-rays (photons) that are then shaped and precisely directed to specific areas within the body.

Local recurrence: Cancer that has recurred (come back) at or near the same place as the original (primary) tumor, usually after a period during which the cancer could not be detected.

Lumpectomy or breast-conserving surgery: An operation to remove a breast cancer and a small amount of surrounding normal tissue, but not the entire breast. Lumpectomy may also be referred to as a partial mastectomy, quadrantectomy, or segmental mastectomy.

Lymphedema: Swelling that results from a blockage in the lymphatic system that prevents lymph fluid from draining normally. Lymphedema occurs most often in an arm or leg that results from the removal of or damage to lymph nodes as a part of cancer treatment.

Macromolecule: A very large molecule, such as a protein, commonly created by the polymerization of smaller subunits and are typically composed of thousands of atoms.

Mammogram: A low-energy X-ray of the breast that is taken with a device that compresses and flattens the breast in order to detect lumps, cysts, or cancers within the breast.

Mammography: The process of using low-energy X-rays to examine the human breast for diagnosis and screening. The goal of mammography is the early detection of breast cancer, typically through detection of characteristic masses or microcalcifications.

Mastectomy: Surgery to remove part or all of the breast; generally, to remove cancerous tissue, although sometimes performed prophylactically to prevent the development of cancer.

Median survival: A statistic that refers to the length of time (in months or years) that half of the patients in a particular group are expected to be alive. In other words, the chance of surviving beyond that time is 50%.

Mediastinum: The area in the mid-chest between the lungs that includes the heart, large veins and arteries, trachea, esophagus, bronchi, and lymph nodes.

Medical dosimetrist: A medical professional who is trained to work alongside a radiation oncologist and certified to develop radiation treatment plans and calculate doses of radiation to cancer patients.

Medical oncologist: A physician trained to diagnose and treat cancer in adults using chemotherapy, hormonal therapy, biological therapy, and targeted therapy.

Medical physicist: A specialist trained in the physics of radiation therapy, x-ray imaging, ultrasound, computed tomography, radiology, nuclear magnetic resonance imaging, and lasers. Medical physicists use a variety of analytical, computer-aided, and bioengineering techniques in their work with patients and with a wide range of medical, technical, and administrative staff.

Metastasis: The spread of cancer cells to new areas of the body, often by way of the lymph system or bloodstream. A metastatic cancer, or metastatic tumor, is one that has spread from the primary site of origin, or where it started, into different areas of the body.

Mohs surgery: A type of surgery that is used for the treatment of skin cancer, especially basal cell or squamous cell carcinoma of the skin. Mohs surgery is a time-consuming process designed to remove all the cancerous tissue in several stages while removing as little of the healthy tissue as possible through the use of microscopic analyses.

MRI (Magnetic Resonance Imaging) scan: A medical scan that produces an image of the body using a strong magnet and radio waves. Unlike other diagnostic imaging tests, an MRI scan can precisely show neurologic tissue (brain, spinal cord, and nerves), muscles, ligaments, tendons, and cartilage.

National Cancer Institute (NCI): A U.S. federal government agency designated for cancer research and training.

NCCN (National Comprehensive Cancer Network): A not-for-profit alliance of 28 leading cancer centers that is devoted to patient care, research, and education, and is dedicated to improving the quality, effectiveness, and efficiency of cancer care.

NCCN guidelines: Widely recognized treatment regimens for the most common cancers that are updated each year by a multidisciplinary group of cancer specialists and used by many oncologists and insurance providers as the standard of care for clinical policies in oncology.

Neoadjuvant chemotherapy: An approach to fighting cancer in which chemotherapy treatments are given before surgery or radiation, usually to shrink the tumor or prevent growth of distant metastasis.

Neurologist: A physician trained to diagnose and treat disorders of the nervous system, including the brain, spinal cord, and nerves.

Neurosurgeon: A physician trained in the surgical treatment of patients with neurological conditions (including tumors) involving the brain, spinal cord, and nerves.

Non-small cell lung cancer (NSCLC): The most common category of lung cancers, which include adenocarcinoma, large cell carcinoma, squamous cell carcinoma, and many others.

NSCLC usually spreads more slowly than small cell lung cancer, but commonly spreads to lymph nodes, lung, liver, bone, and brain.

NRG Oncology: One of five U.S. network groups of the NCI National Clinical Trials Network (NCTN) Program. NRG formed from the merger of the National Surgical Adjuvant Breast and Bowel Project (NSABP), the Radiation Therapy Oncology Group (RTOG), and the Gynecological Oncology Group (GOG). It is a non-profit research organization formed to conduct oncologic clinical research and to broadly disseminate study results for informing clinical decision-making and healthcare policy.

Nurse practitioners (NP): An Advanced Practice Provider (APP), or mid-level provider, that is a registered nurse (RN) who has completed an advanced training program in a medical specialty and may be a primary, direct healthcare provider that can prescribe most medications.

Oligometastasis: A type of cancer spread whereby cancer cells travel from the original (primary) site of tumor to a small number of new areas (typically up to five metastatic tumors) in other parts of the body. Patients with oligometastasis generally fare better than patients with more numerous metastasis and may be candidates for SBRT or surgery, in addition to chemotherapy and/or immunotherapy.

Oncogenes: A gene that has the potential to cause cancer and is often mutated or expressed at high levels in tumor cells.

Oncologic surgery: A type of surgery to completely remove (cut out) a tumor or cancer while being careful not to contaminate or spread cancer cells to surrounding normal tissues by maintaining a small, continuous shell of healthy tissue around the tumor, called an en-bloc resection. Oncologic surgeries also usually include a lymph node dissection and/or sampling of any suspicious tissues at the time of surgery.

Palliative radiation: Radiation treatments to shrink a cancer, slow down its growth, or control symptoms caused by a cancer. Since the goal is not to cure the cancer, lower doses of radiation may be used to relieve or prevent symptoms of cancer growth and improve quality of life while minimizing the risk of side effects.

Pathologic staging: A method that uses the microscopic findings from a pathology report following a surgery or lymph node dissection to more precisely describe how much cancer is in a cancer patient's body by defining where the original tumor is located, how big it is, if it has spread, and to where it has spread. Pathologic staging may be slightly different from and is *more* accurate than simple clinical staging (from medical scans) because of the additional information obtained from surgery.

Pathology report: A report to describe the microscopic findings from a pathologist regarding the cells and tissues resulting from a biopsy or surgery that are often used to make a diagnosis of cancer or other disease.

PEG (Percutaneous Endoscopic Gastrostomy) tube: A feeding tube that is passed into a patient's stomach through the abdominal wall and is a common way to provide feeding when oral intake is not adequate or possible.

PET (Positron Emission Tomography) scan: A medical scan in which a small amount of radioactive glucose (sugar) is injected into a vein, and a scanner is used to make computerized pictures of areas inside the body where the glucose is taken up. Since cancer cells often consume more glucose the normal cells, PET scans are used to locate groups of cancer cells in the body. Caution: Since many body tissues and processes, areas of trauma, and infections also consume glucose, uptake may not always represent cancer and results must be interpreted by a trained physician.

PET/CT scan: A medical scan that combines a PET scanner and a CT scanner into one machine to combine the data from both and obtain more detailed images of areas inside the body. A PET-CT scan is primarily used to more precisely locate groups of cancer cells to aid in clinical staging, treatment planning, or assess the effectiveness of a cancer treatment. Caution: Since PET scans rely on glucose uptake and many body tissues and processes, areas of trauma, and infections also consume glucose, uptake may not always represent cancer and results must be interpreted by a trained physician.

Physician's assistant (PA): An Advanced Practice Provider (APP), or mid-level provider, that is specially trained and certified to provide basic medical services (such as the diagnosis and treatment of common ailments) usually under the supervision of a licensed physician and can prescribe most medications.

Port: A surgically implanted catheter that is placed under the skin of the upper chest, also called a venous port or central venous catheter, that is used to access a patient's bloodstream through which blood can be withdrawn or medications injected. A port may be left in place for many weeks to months and helps decrease the need to have repeated and uncomfortable blood draws or injections from a peripheral vein in the arm or extremity.

Postoperative radiation therapy: Radiation treatments given after a surgery.

Primary brain tumor: A cancer that starts in the brain by forming from brain cells, the membranes around the brain (meninges), nerves, or glands.

Prostate seed implant or prostate brachytherapy: A highly effective form of radiation therapy used to treat prostate cancer that involves placing small radioactive "seeds" in the prostate gland near cancer cells while sparing surrounding normal tissues from excess doses of radiation.

Proton therapy or proton beam therapy: A type of radiation therapy that uses high-energy protons (positively charged subatomic particles) rather than X-rays to destroy cancer cells. While the delivery of high-dose radiation and effectiveness of proton therapy has been shown to be equivalent to traditional X-ray therapy, some argue that the benefit of proton therapy is a decrease in the very low dose region of radiation delivered to some surrounding normal tissues, which may further reduce the risk of secondary cancers, particularly in children.

PSA (Prostate Specific Antigen): A protein that is produced by the prostate gland in men and can be measured via a blood test that is used to screen for cancer of the prostate and to monitor treatment of disease. PSA levels naturally rise as a man ages due to natural prostate enlargement, but rapid rises often indicate the formation or presence of prostate cancer cells.

PSA progression: The steady increase in the amount of prostate specific antigen found in the blood on test results.

Quality-of-life: The patient's ability to enjoy normal life activities.

Radiation-induced secondary malignancies (RISM) or secondary cancer: A new and different cancer that occurs in an individual as a result of previous cancer treatments. RISM occur within a previous radiation-field while secondary malignancies may result from either radiation or chemotherapy months or years after treatment.

Radiation necrosis: A potential long-term central nervous system (CNS) complication of radiotherapy or radiosurgery indicating damage to normal cells of the brain or spinal cord that most commonly presents with edema (swelling), enhancement on MRI, and symptoms of increased intracranial pressure. Note: Radiation necrosis mimics tumor recurrence on most medical scans and may require a biopsy or resection to differentiate.

Radiation oncologist: A physician and cancer specialist trained to diagnose, stage, and treat many different types of cancer using various forms of radiation (x-rays, electrons, protons, brachytherapy, etc.)

Radiation therapy (radiotherapy): A type of cancer treatment that uses ionizing (high-energy) radiation treatments (usually X-rays) to precisely target and kill cancer cells while attempting to minimize side effects from surrounding normal tissues.

Radiation therapy technologists (RTTs) or RT technicians: Healthcare professionals specially trained to deliver radiation treatments to patients with cancer and other diseases. RTTs maintain and operate radiation machines, ensure that safety procedures are followed properly, keep records, and monitor patients during their radiation treatments.

Radiation therapist: See radiation therapy technologist.

Radical prostatectomy: A surgical procedure performed by a urologist that removes the entire prostate gland and some surrounding tissue. Prostatectomy may include a pelvic lymph node dissection and may be performed via an open procedure or laparoscopically, either manually or robotically.

Radiosensitizer: Any substance that makes tumor cells easier to kill with radiation therapy and includes different classes of medicines, particularly chemotherapies such as cisplatin, 5-Fluorouracil, gemcitabine, etc.

Research trials (clinical trials): Research investigations in which people volunteer to test new treatments, interventions, or tests to prevent, detect, treat or manage various diseases or medical conditions.

Resectable: Able to be removed (resected) by surgery.

Screening tests: A test or study that is not considered diagnostic (i.e. not used to evaluate a patient's symptoms), but rather is used on a large group or population in order to identify a subset of persons who should have additional testing to determine the presence or absence of a disease.

Sentinel lymph node biopsy: A staging procedure that uses a special blue dye and/or a radioactive isotope to examine the first lymph node that receives lymphatic drainage from a tumor to see if cancer cells have spread to the lymph nodes.

Side effects: In medicine, a side effect is an effect, whether therapeutic or adverse, that is secondary to the one intended.

Squamous cell carcinoma: Also called epidermoid carcinoma, they are cancers formed from the flat, thin cells of the skin, the lining of the digestive tract, respiratory tract, or hollow organs. They are the most common type of cancer of the anus, cervix, head and neck, and vagina.

Small cell lung cancer (SCLC): A type of lung cancer in which the cells appear small and round under the microscope, previously called oat cell lung cancer, and is an aggressive (fast growing) cancer that often spreads to lymph nodes and through the blood to other parts of the lung, liver, brain, bone, etc.

Stereotactic Body Radiation Therapy (SBRT): An advanced form of radiation therapy, also known as Stereotactic ABlative Radiotherapy (SABR), uses computer optimization and Image-Guided Radiation Therapy to precisely deliver very high doses of radiation in 2-5 fractions to small tumors with minimal side effects and high rates of local control.

Stereotactic Radiosurgery (SRS): A nonsurgical, advanced form of radiation therapy that is delivered in one fraction and used to treat functional abnormalities and small tumors of the brain with very precise, high-dose radiation with minimal side effects and high rates of local control.

Surgery: The branch of medicine that involves cutting, abrading, suturing, or otherwise physically changing body tissues and organs during an operation to treat disease or injury.

Surgical margin or resection margin: The edge or margin of a specimen of tissue that was surgically removed during an operation and is evaluated under a microscope by a pathologist to determine if cancer cells extend up to the line of resection. A positive surgical margin indicates that some cancer cells remain within the patient, while the more favorable, negative surgical margins indicate that all the cancer cells visible under the microscope were successfully removed at the area of the surgery.

Three-dimensional (3D) breast tomography (tomosynthesis): A medical scan that is a new type of digital mammogram which uses X-rays to create both 2-dimensional and 3-dimensional images of the breast to screen for and identify breast cancer.

TORS (transoral robotic surgery): A surgery that uses a robot arm with attached camera to give the surgeon a 3-dimensional (3D) image that enables better removal of cancers from hard-to-reach areas of the mouth and throat.

Transcribe or transcription: A biologic process that occurs within the nucleus of all living cells by which information from DNA is copied into RNA and is subsequently used to construct proteins and other molecules necessary for life.

Tumor markers: A substance that can be detected in higher-than-normal amounts in the blood, urine, or body tissues of some patients with certain types of cancer. A tumor marker may be produced by a tumor (cancer) itself, or by the body as a response to the tumor. They can be used to screen patients for the presence of some cancers or to monitor the effectiveness of some cancer treatments, but there are still no reliable tumor markers for many types of cancers. Examples include CA-125 for ovarian cancer, CEA for colon-type cancers, and PSA for prostate cancer.

Ultrasound: A medical scan, also called sonography, that uses high-frequency sound waves to produce images of structures within your body. Ultrasound has limited applications to certain parts of the body but does not use X-rays nor isotopes and is completely safe.

Vaginal cuff brachytherapy: A type of radiation treatment used to deliver very localized doses of radiation to the upper part of the vagina following a hysterectomy for cervical or uterine cancer. Radiation is delivered a few times per week over several treatments via a small, hollow applicator (plastic tube or cylinder) placed within the vaginal canal by a radiation oncologist.

Volumetric Modulated Arc Therapy (VMAT): An advanced form of radiation treatment which uses only one or two machine rotations of a linear accelerator around a patient to quickly deliver highly-shaped doses of radiation with improved tumor coverage and sparing of normal tissues compared with conventional radiotherapy techniques.

World Health Organization (WHO): The specialized agency of the United Nations that is concerned with international public health.

X-ray treatment: A type of radiation therapy that uses high-energy radiation from photons (i.e. X-rays), typically from linear accelerators, to kill cancer cells and shrink tumors.

ABOUT THE AUTHOR

Dr. Plants is a cancer specialist who lives in Charleston, West Virginia, with his wife and three children. He graduated *summa cum laude* with a bachelor's in chemistry and with a doctorate in medicine from West Virginia University prior to completing a medical residency in radiation oncology from the University of Alabama at Birmingham in 2004. He returned to his hometown, where he has practiced oncology for the past 15 years and cared for thousands of cancer patients. He has treated all types of cancer, including—brain, head and neck, lung, breast, gastrointestinal, genitourinary, and gynecologic cancers. He is also skilled at stereotactic radiosurgery, brachytherapy, Image-Guided (IGRT), Intensity-Modulated (IMRT/VMAT), and Stereotactic Body Radiation Therapy (SBRT) for a variety of cancers. Dr. Plants also actively participates in his community through multiple local charities and enjoys speaking at local schools, churches, and conferences.

NOTES

PART ONE

Chapter 2

<u>1</u> https://www.cancer.gov/publications/dictionaries/cancer-terms

Chapter 4

<u>1</u> Sun, J., et al., J Invest Surg. 2012 Feb; 25(1):33-6.

<u>2</u> Kim, AW., et al., Semin Thorac Cardiovasc Surg. 2009 Winter; 21(4):298-308.

Chapter 5

<u>1</u> Chow, F., Colorectal liver metastases: An update on multidisciplinary approach. World J Hepatol. 2019 Feb 27; 11(2): 150-172.

<u>2</u> Greco, C., Phenotype-Oriented Ablation of Oligometastatic Cancer with Single Dose Radiation Therapy. Int J of Rad Onc Biol Phys. 2019 Jul 1; 104(3): 593-603.

<u>3</u> Horning, S., 50 Years in Hematology, Ch. 2. The Cure of Hodgkin's Lymphoma, pp. 16-17, 2008.

Chapter 9

1 John Ng et al., Cancer Manag Res. 2015; 7: 1–11.

2 Hall, E. et al., Intensity-modulated radiation therapy, protons, and the risk of second cancers. Int J Radiat Oncol Biol Phys. 2006; 65:1–7.

3 1990 Recommendations of the International Commission on Radiological Protection. Ann ICRP. 1991; 21:1–201.

Chapter 13

1 Hughes, K., et al., Lumpectomy plus tamoxifen with or without irradiation in women age 70 years or older with early breast cancer: long-term follow-up of CALGB 9343. J Clin Oncol, 31(19), July 2013; 2382-7.

Chapter 14

1 The Harris Poll from July 10-August 10, 2018 among 4,887 U.S. adults ages 18 and older. https://www.asco.org/about-asco/press-center/news-releases/national-survey-reveals-surprising-number-americans-believe

2 Skyler, B., et al., Use of Alternative Medicine for Cancer and Its Impact on Survival. J Nat Cancer Institute, 110(1), January 2018; 121–124.

3 Bhavani S., et al., Prevalence and Survival Impact of Pretreatment Cancer-Associated Weight Loss: A Tool for Guiding Early Palliative Care. J of Oncology Practice, April 2018; e238–e250.

PART TWO

Chapter 2

1 Hughes, K., et al., Lumpectomy plus tamoxifen with or without irradiation in women age 70 years or older with early breast cancer: long-term follow-up of CALGB 9343. J Clin Oncol, 31(19), July 2013; 2382-7.

2 Kunkler, I., et al., Breast-conserving surgery with or without irradiation in women aged 65 years or older with early breast cancer (PRIME II): a randomised controlled trial. The Lancet, 16(3), March 2015; 266-273.

Made in United States
North Haven, CT
03 December 2021

11905096R00098